Smoke Rings

When everyone tells you not to but you want to anyway.

1st Edition

Eli Camp, ND, DHANP, VNMI

with contributions by Amanda Blandford, ND, LMT

The information in this book is intended as an educational reference only, not as medical advice. The information provided is designed to help you make informed decisions and is not intended as a substitute for medical treatment or to go against your doctor's recommendations. Information provided in this book is not a guarantee of any type of outcome. The authors and publisher disclaim any liability in connection with the use of the information contained within this book.

2024 by Eli Camp, ND

All rights reserved. No part of this book may be reproduced or transmitted in any form or by any means, electronic or mechanical, including photocopying, recording, or any other information storage and retrieval system, without the written permission of the publisher.

Published in 2024 by
Vital Health Publishing, LLC
Tahlequah, Oklahoma

Printed in the United States of America

Book Design by Juan Carlos Martin Cobano, www.setelee.com

Cover Design by Antonio Conway

ISBN: 978-0-9995165-9-1

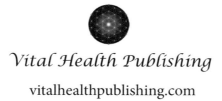

To my family, big Brian, Brian Michael, and Sophia, thank you for the kind of love that allows me to be all of who I am.

Table of Contents

Acknowledgements .... *VII*
Foreword .... *IX*
Introduction .... *XI*

Chapter 1: The Vitalistic Approach to Health 1
Chapter 2: Creating the Healthiest Version of You 7
Chapter 3: The Basics – Good Medicine for Everyone 10
Chapter 4: A Tour of Natural Therapies 22
Chapter 5: A Tour of the Smoker's Body 38
Chapter 6: The Air We Breathe 45
Chapter 7: The Blood Running Through Our Veins 57
Chapter 8: Our Internal Detoxification 67
Chapter 9: Our Reproductive Parts 81
Chapter 10: Windows to the World 96
Chapter 11: Beauty is Not Just Skin Deep 109
Chapter 12: Wipeout! 120
Chapter 13: Keeping Your Metabolism on Track 134
Chapter 14: The Mental and Emotional You 141
Chapter 15: The Smoldering Nerves 147
Chapter 16: What About The Gut? 155
Chapter 17: Bones and Muscles 164
Chapter 18: The Master Reset: Sleep 172

Chapter 19: Your Defenses 180
Chapter 20: The Apothecary 187
A Smoker's Daily Plan *206*
Closing Thoughts *210*
Resources *211*
References *213*
Image Attributions *239*
About the Author *240*
Other books by Vital Health Publishing *242*

Acknowledgements

First, I would like to thank Dr. Amanda Blandford who did a wonderful job compiling the research for this book and for her help finding the right words. I am not sure how long this project would have taken without her efforts. I am grateful for Dr. Judith Thompson, a friend, colleague, and business partner who loves almost all of my ideas and helps me brainstorm to bring the most promising ones to life. Hats off to my graphic designer, and eldest son, Tony Conway; this book is beautiful. And, a special thanks to Alex and Luka for their support, ideas, and help to bring this book to the world.

I appreciate my many colleagues who listened to the idea of this book and only offered encouragement, boosting my confidence in the idea that others might need this resource.

There are so many teachers and mentors who have each played a part in sculpting my perception of life, health, myself, and how to be a healer. The first person who convinced me I could learn anything I desired was Dr. Doug Gaffin whom I met in 1995 during my first semester of college. When I met him, he was the head of scorpion research at OU and took me under his wing. While all my instructors had an impact, Drs. Stephen Messer, Thomas Kruzel, Jared Zeff, and Letitia Dick profoundly influenced how I practice medicine. For that, I am forever grateful. I would also like to thank James Sensenig, ND (1948-2019) who showed me a new paradigm of life and medicine; without that knowledge, I would have written a much different book.

Finally, a heartfelt thanks to my husband Brian, daughter Sophia, and son Brian Michael who have supported me through many long days and nights while I put this book together.

Foreword

Dr. Camp has done it again by creating a book powerful in its simplicity. This book is designed to reach smokers, people who have been ostracized by the general public, in ways other texts fail to do. Decades ago smoking was a massive status symbol and everyone was doing it, including the doctors who told their patients how to deal with illness and disease. It's still possible to find black-and-white images online with doctors smiling as they take a drag.

Over the last few decades in the United States, smokers have been declining in number. This can be partly attributed to educating young people about the potential harm of smoking, often preventing them from smoking in the first place. There are now medications and patches to help wean smokers off of cigarettes, in addition to better programs created to walk people through the process of quitting. As a result, today's smokers are constantly exposed to the negative effects of smoking. They are told it's a bad habit, you're killing yourself, etc. One of the first things most modern doctors will tell their patients is to quit smoking, but what about the smoker? What about those who know it's terrible, but aren't ready to quit? Is there a way for them to be healthier?

This book answers this question in a well-thought-out manner. First, consider this: the cardiovascular system, including the heart and all the blood vessels in the body, is very susceptible to damage from smoking. The damage is not limited to just cigarette smoking. Over 4,000 years ago in ancient Egypt, people also died from cardiovascular disease. Scientists did CT scans of 137 mummies and discovered probable or definite atherosclerosis in roughly one-third of them. It is also known that smoke exposure to everything from wildfires to being around a wood-burning cooking stove for a couple of hours raises blood pressure slightly. Between the oxidative stress, impact on the autonomic nervous system, and inhaled chemicals, this can spell disaster over time. Now that you know all smoke harms you, what's the big deal about smoking cigarettes? This book will answer this question and more.

If you are a smoker, you may already be thinking this is another one of those books putting you down for smoking. This couldn't be farther from the truth. As a Naturopathic doctor, I believe health is possible for everyone. Of course, not smoking is the best health option, but what's most important is deciding what is best for you. Smoking may be something you enjoy doing with friends, it may be a simple stress reliever that has grown into a habit, or it may be the only thing you see as holding your life together. Whatever your story and reason, it's up to you to decide who you are and how you want to live your life.

If you are a healthcare provider, you may also be wondering how this book would be useful for you. You went through medical school, and you've stayed up-to-date on the research, but stop and think: how often were smokers specifically addressed? Have you been frustrated working with smokers who won't quit? Most doctors, myself included, go into medicine to help people, and sometimes the quit smoking speech doesn't achieve the effect you'd want. Here at your fingertips is an approach that presents options you may not have considered as well as reasons why they may be helpful for your patients.

Now, this book is specifically written for nicotine smokers, but the concepts apply to many types of inhaled substances including herbs (damiana, mugwort, mullein, etc.), marijuana, and tobacco. This book is for those who are looking for health whether they are a chain smoker, a social smoker, or a former smoker. There's something in here for you to learn and apply to your life. Whether or not you are ready to quit, this book is a judgment-free place for you to learn how to be your healthiest self. Even if you are too busy to read it from cover to cover, the thoughtful design of this book helps guide you so you can pick and choose what's most useful to you.

If you are a smoker, were a smoker, know smokers, or work with smokers, this book will definitely speak to you.

Dr. Amanda Blandford
Naturopathic Doctor,
Licensed Massage Therapist

INTRODUCTION

Why this book?

When I was 11 years old, and living in Penfield, Illinois, population 550, the only place to hang out was the grain elevator in the middle of town. Across the street was the local pub and post office.

Every morning before school, I would meet with a few of the other sixth graders at the grain elevator, which doubled as the bus stop for the high schoolers. Together, each of us would suck down two or three smokes from the manager's desk drawer before getting on the bus. There was a concrete wall to hide behind and the elevator manager was kind enough to buy a carton of smokes at a time so we could buy our packs from him. Sometimes, we would stop by for a quick one after school—but that was risky. We might carry the smell home for our parents to notice.

We did not think about smoking and how it affected our health. At the time most of our parents smoked. Besides, if it was that bad, why would they do it? As children, we did not think about lung damage, COPD or emphysema, early wrinkles, yellow skin and nails, our blood vessels, brain, liver, or any of those things. We were the cool kids, hanging out with the high schoolers; not to mention, we were exhilarated to fool our parents.

None of us knew that the path from having a few smokes a day to a life-long addiction was a *very* short trip.

Today, there is an incredible body of research and knowledge about the effects of smoking on the human body. There is just as much, if not more, information regarding strategies to help people quit smoking. Pharmaceutical companies have even jumped on board this lucrative quit-smoking train and produced prescription drugs designed to help the body overcome the physical addiction to tobacco. Unfortunately, many of those products have side effects as severe as smoking itself. In some cases, the side effects are much worse.

Doctors are usually the first to say, "Quit smoking! Your blood pressure is elevated, your lung function is decreased; the most important thing you can do is quit!" While it is true that quitting is the best thing you can do for yourself, I find myself asking a different question. Aside from quitting, is there anything a person who chooses to smoke can do to be healthier? This question stuck with me, and so I went looking. I believe each person has as much right as the other to choose a lifestyle, partners, work, and beliefs, and there are people who choose to smoke. I also believe each and every person can do something every day to create greater health, yes, even for people who smoke.

Forty-five years after I first asked the question, the doctor in me has to agree that quitting is the BEST thing to do. My father died the year I started medical school. He smoked three packs a day his entire life beginning at age fourteen. He likely had his last smoke a few hours before he died. I have always wondered if I knew then what I know now if I could have helped him live a longer life. You see, it turns out there is a lot you can do while you are (or are not) on the journey to quit. When you smoke (anything), you introduce poisons into your body. These poisons damage every cell, which in turn, creates a pull on the *vis medicatrix naturae*—the innate healing ability within each of us. The body wants to be healthy and when there is something out of balance it tries to self-correct, to heal. When the body is healing there are symptoms and when there are no longer symptoms, there is nothing left for it to heal.

When we use the laws of nature to assist the body in healing itself, healing happens. When we use the laws of nature to oppose the body, disease happens. It is that simple.

You may be wondering what the end of the story is for that eleven-year-old sitting by the side of that grain elevator. Well, I can tell you it is a happy ending with smoking left far behind. If smoking was good for me I would still happily enjoy a smoke after dinner, or with a tasty cup of coffee. But, it isn't good for me or you. Instead of focusing on the obvious, I want to focus on how to create a healthier version of yourself, something I wish I could have done for my father.

What I hope this book will do for you.

The intention of this book is to help smokers of any substance learn how to support, protect, and heal their body as much as possible on a regular basis. The amount of research on the effects of tobacco is staggering. Wherever possible we have included what is relevant for other smokable materials. Much of the information presented in this book is not limited to smokers but can be used by anyone seeking to better their overall health.

I hope this book gives you a sense of wholeness about your body. As you read, I will try to help you understand how each part of the body affects the others and teach you how to support yours every day to create for you a better state of health. I look forward to how you will use the information from this book to establish new practices and habits to support your body and its healing.

The best way to use this book.

Readers, friends, I ask that you spend time reading "Chapter 1: The Vitalistic Approach to Health" as it sets the foundation of the perspective I teach from, believe in, and practice from daily. It's best to read through the book in its entirety before you begin modifying your health choices. This book has been designed for those who are pinched for time and unable to read from cover to cover. Chapters 1-5 are critical to understanding this text as a whole. Once you finish those chapters you can pick and choose what's most important to you and your goals. You will find examples and suggestions throughout the book on how to make potential changes, but ultimately you are the boss and are in charge of deciding how this information fits best into your life. I believe that health is not a right or privilege; rather, it is a responsibility we owe ourselves and those around us. Finally, I ask you to share this book with others looking to improve their lives and overall health.

Chapter 1:
The Vitalistic Approach to Health

Vitalism

Humans of the 21st century have come a long way over the last 5,000 years in their understanding of the world, the environment, and the biology of life. As new information is discovered, it will enter into the collective knowledge of humankind and be accessible to those who openly seek to find it. This knowledge can give us the least toxic and most current health-building strategies for both humans and the planet. When it comes to the ever-evolving body of knowledge about human health we can find many perspectives and approaches to preventing death, sustaining life, and creating health.

One perspective is Vitalism. This approach to health is founded on the understanding there are chemical, physical, and energetic forces at work around and within all living beings. These forces affect humans as well as everything else in our collective environment. Each of these forces on its own can create an effect (something that is observable) but in combination, they far exceed the individual effects adding up to a more powerful change. There are many examples of this within nature, chemistry, and physics. One example from grade school is a homemade volcano. This uses baking soda, vinegar, and a tube, usually made of clay or plastic. When you combine the soda and vinegar in the bottom of the tube, they erupt as spectacular foam lava. The effect is far greater than either baking soda or vinegar could produce on its own, in effect creating synergy between the two when combined.

The Vitalist understands humans are part of an interconnected system in which forces act in a synergistic manner. There is an energetic force within all beings and although it does not have a direct definition in Western terms, it is known as *Qi* in Chinese medicine and *prana* in Ayurvedic medicine. In Naturopathic medicine, this energetic force is known as the *Vis* or the Vital Force. Together, various biological, chemical, and energetic forces create vitality and drive normal, healthy function within the body. The concept of *Vis* is important. To explain it another way, it means the body is always on autopilot trying to be its most healthy. The force that drives healing in all living systems is known as the *Vis Medicatrix Naturae*, or the healing power of nature. When something blocks or prevents the body from doing what it does naturally, imbalance occurs and symptoms of illness and disease can be observed.

In Vitalism, the body is viewed as a living organism rather than a machine with replaceable parts. Our body is much more than the sum of its pieces and parts. When damaged, a machine cannot repair itself. Our body, in contrast, has an innate intelligence that guides healing and restoration. Vitalism recognizes and engages this intelligence or "body wisdom" to speed recovery from illness and build even greater levels of health.

The Vis

The word *Vis* is defined as a force or a power. When looking at a person's level of health, there are specific characteristics and traits that indicate whether the *Vis* is thriving. People sometimes think of this as "vitality", which is often defined as physical or mental vigor, especially when highly developed. There are characteristics and traits which indicate vitality—the state of the *Vis* that flows through us and in us. The following are all characteristics of a strong *Vis*:

- Bright eyes
- Clear skin
- A robust complexion
- Strong nails and hair
- Toned muscles
- Enduring energy
- Sound sleep
- Strong digestion
- Daily bowel movements
- A stable, predominantly optimistic mood
- Good cognitive function

When a person is sick, the observable features of a strong *Vis* are missing or weakened. Unless the *Vis* is restored symptoms of illness will appear sooner or later. Sometimes symptoms appear immediately as they do in acute illness or injury, and other times they develop over weeks, months, and even years. Regardless of when symptoms appear, characteristics of a weak *Vis* might be:

- Dull eyes
- Rough and dry skin

- A pale complexion
- Weak nails and thinning hair
- Soft muscles
- Lack of energy
- Poor and disturbed sleep
- Disturbed digestion
- Irregular bowel movements
- Unstable moods
- Poor cognitive function

There are many ways for poor vitality, or a weak *Vis,* to exhibit in people. If vitality is not restored, the body has difficulty healing and at some point, it cannot recover. Without recovery, death is the result. In "Chapter 3: The Basics - Good Medicine for Everyone," the core areas of basic health are discussed; all areas of basic health are intricately intertwined and can produce a strong and thriving *Vis.*

The Guiding Principles

Every profession on this planet is guided by principles and Naturopathic medicine is no different. The following principles are central to this practice of medicine.

The Healing Power of Nature (*Vis Medicatrix Naturae*)

The natural state of the body is to try to be healthy. When one looks at nature, the inherent capacity for healing can be observed. Wounds heal, fractures mend, pastures regenerate, animals recover, and new growth appears. Left to its own processes, the body's default state is to always move toward health. The main objectives of the Naturopathic doctor are to support the healing process of nature by:

- Giving the body what it needs
- Moving toxicity out of the body
- Restoring the composition of blood and lymph
- Stimulating the natural healing ability of each person

First Do No Harm (*Primum Non Nocere*)

Before a Naturopathic doctor does anything, they must first do no harm. This means that with every therapy, lifestyle change, vitamin, supplement, herb, or activity, the person a Naturopathic doctor is treating must walk away in a better state of health than when they arrived.

Find and Treat the Underlying Cause (*Tolle Causam*)

There is always a reason why the body shows symptoms of illness.

Before treatment can begin, one has to know what the underlying cause of illness or disease is. Only then can an individualized, health-restoring, treatment plan be put together. A treatment plan is designed to remove what should not be there, add what is missing, and slowly but gently move the person from illness to wellness in a safe, gentle, and non-toxic manner. The most effective doctor educates their patients about why they are doing what they are doing and how the chosen course of action is helpful.

Doctor as Teacher (*Docere*)

Doctor comes from the word "*Docere*" which means teacher. A doctor's highest calling is to teach a person what will keep them well and what will make them unwell. While a person's state of health is ultimately up to them, it is a doctor's job to give their patients the knowledge they need to build health.

Hippocrates, the father of all branches of medicine, said

> "It is thus with regard to the disease called Sacred: it appears to me to be nowise more divine nor more sacred than other diseases, but has a natural cause from the originates like other affections. Men regard its nature and cause as divine from ignorance and wonder...."
> – Hippocrates, *On the Sacred Disease*

This means that until a person is taught the true nature of disease, they are unable to change the course of their state of health. It is up to the doctor to teach their patient what their body is capable of and how to achieve their highest potential.

Treat the Whole Person (*Tolle Totum*)

Each human being is so much more than the sum of their individual parts, as is their health at any given moment. From the moment a human is born everything eaten, breathed, thought, seen, and felt starts to shape their lifelong health experience. When it is time for a doctor to help fix things that have gone wrong, the entire being must be looked at and put back into balance. A doctor must look at the emotional, spiritual, and physical states to help each patient regain the balance that will lead to their optimal health.

Prevention is the Best Cure (*Prevenire*)

Even though the body is an incredible masterpiece, one capable of regenerating and healing, not everything that goes wrong with the body can be fixed. A person can be made more comfortable, pain can be eased, and a chronic condition can be managed, but once enough damage has occurred, it may not be possible to completely restore the body's function. Thankfully, most illnesses (not all) can be prevented with proper diet, a healthy mindset, exercise, proper hydration, a supportive environment, and proper supplements.

Health can be improved at any stage of life, so it is never too late to begin a journey of well-being. What a person does today will impact their health tomorrow. It is important to ask yourself in all that you do—does this create health or disease? As humans demand a healthier environment, healthier food, and the removal of poisons from the water and air, the earth itself will begin to heal.

The Journey

Absolute illness and absolute health still end in death. That is the cycle of all life on this planet. From a vitalistic perspective, getting healthy is not about avoiding death; instead, it is about traveling through your life in the healthiest state possible. It is about the day-to-day journey and discovery of self. Instead, you should focus on the choices you have every day and the knowledge of how to create health within your body. This allows each human to reach their highest potential, enjoy a life free of the symptoms of illness, and prevent dependence on the medical system to live an independent life far into old age. The journey is about experiencing healthfulness for as much of your life as possible.

When it comes to the vitalistic approach of medicine and the activity of smoking, the goal is to support the body, mind, and spirit. There is an entire arsenal of tools, therapies, and strategies that can help you on the path to becoming a healthier version of yourself. Be gentle with yourself as you journey and take it one day and one choice at a time. Come back to these pages again and again, chapter by chapter, until you have put strategies and habits in place that can help you end each day healthier than how you began.

Chapter 2:
Creating the Healthiest Version of You

Sayings such as, "Prevention is the best medicine," or "An ounce of prevention is worth a pound of cure" are common. These phrases carry the message that there is great value in staying healthy. That it is better to become and remain as healthy as possible and avoid any other kind of medicine. Thankfully, there are habits to practice every day to keep yourself and your loved ones in good health. Keeping up these habits will require time and effort, but will promote your quality of life, allow you to pursue the things you love, and to live independently well into your elder years. The body knows how to be and stay healthy. Doing things that build or restore and then maintain wellness keeps your body in good health. But what does the healthiest version of you look like?

The Spectrum of Health

Health can be understood as a spectrum. On one end of the spectrum is the best possible health with extreme sickness, and often premature death, at the other end. In between these extremes are varying levels of health and sickness. Most people are not trying to create their healthiest possible state; they are simply trying to find a place where they are "healthy enough" and this looks different for each person.

What is healthy enough? The symptoms of illness begin long before a diagnosis is made and even longer before people reach their most unwell state. The opposite is also true—as someone becomes healthier, symptoms of illness begin to disappear long before they reach their greatest level of wellness. Another way to think about this is, when your body becomes healthy enough, symptoms of illness begin to disappear.

The next chapter contains the basics of building health, but before that, it is important to understand how everyone has a different capacity or potential for health. This capacity is not set in stone. There are many factors when determining someone's health potential. Factors such as lifestyle, genetics, environment, knowledge, resources, and social groups can all influence health as well as what people are taught by their caregivers. People begin learning about health and illness from the moment they are born. Caregivers teach their children how to eat, exercise, sleep, and live in particular ways. This includes the kind of food eaten, the purity of the water drank, the quality of the air breathed, and other factors such as the way people speak to one another, the type of exercise or non-exercise that is done, the kind of friends to keep, the media watched or listened to, and much more. Sometimes, the lifestyle people are taught does not build health. For instance, take a person who has a genetic predisposition to diabetes and add to that a toxic environment, insufficient knowledge, a lack of resources, and the teachings of an unhealthy lifestyle, you have someone who has a lower potential for health.

Some people figure out early in life that they are capable of and have a desire to be healthier. To fulfill that desire, a person must make a conscious choice to change how they approach health. They must learn how to do things differently and use that knowledge to change their potential, to increase their capacity for health.

The Signs of Health

When you hear "The Signs of Health", what comes to mind? The Oxford English dictionary defines health as "the state of being free from symptoms of illness or injury." If health is defined as "free from symptoms of illness" then this means that the majority of people who are not currently experiencing any symptoms of disease are healthy. In this scenario, a person who has 80% blockage in the main arteries of their heart and no outward symptoms could be considered healthy! This person may be on the verge of a heart attack but is regarded as healthy because there are currently no symptoms of illness. For all practical purposes, this definition seems faulty.

Instead, let's consider this definition from Merriam-Webster: Health is "the condition of being sound in body, mind or spirit; especially freedom from physical disease or pain." This allows health to be understood as a continuum, one in which a person can move in any direction and be more or less healthy, based on the decisions they make. Decisions about the way to eat, live, and think move a person either a step toward or a step away from health.

Much like the symptoms of illness apparent when the *Vis* is strong or weak, there are signs when a person is healthy. These will vary from person to person, and the healthier a person is the more signs will be present. In general, the signs of health are:

- Pain-free state including movement, digestion, elimination, and sleep
- Energy that lasts the day

- Deep and refreshing sleep
- Clear and balanced thoughts
- Optimism and creativity
- Ability to breathe
- A digestive system that breaks down nutrients taken in and distributes them to the body
- Normal blood pressure and blood sugar regulation
- Regular bowel movements and urination
- Clear and radiant skin

Keeping this list in mind, when it comes to smoking, what is healthy enough? A good place to start is to review the basics of building health.

Chapter 3:
The Basics – Good Medicine for Everyone

Since the 1600s, doctors and other people within the practice of medicine have used the term "hygiene" when discussing the basic health practices of a person. Although today, it is common to define hygiene as how clean someone is, that is just one facet of its definition; hygiene is all that makes up the health practices of a person.

Dr. Samuel Hahnemann, one of the greatest teachers of medicine, is the only physician to have a statue in the United States capital. He wrote the *Organon of Medicine,* one of the first books I read in medical school over twenty years ago. I continue to read it at least once every year to keep myself grounded in a clear understanding of health and disease. The first thing he wrote in this book, the most important thing for a physician to remember above all else, is:

> "The physician's high and only mission is to restore the sick to health, to cure, as it is termed."
> –Dr. Samuel Hahnemann, 1810

He also spoke about a person's health practices and taught that if hygiene was not in order then a doctor could not diagnose someone with a chronic disease. In paragraph 77 of the *Organon*, he instructs physicians:

> "Diseases engendered by prolonged exposure to avoidable noxious influences should not be called chronic."

In other words, diseases that can be brought about by the following should not be considered chronic.

- Habitual indulgence in harmful food or drink
- All kinds of excesses that undermine health
- Prolonged deprivation of things necessary to life
- Unhealthy places, especially swampy regions
- Dwelling only in cellars, damp workplaces, or other closed quarters
- Lack of exercise or fresh air
- Physical or mental overexertion
- Continuing emotional stress

Dr. Hahnemann's words stress that before a doctor determines someone has a chronic disease, there are many things to take into consideration. For example, how they eat, sleep, exercise, play, live, their environment, etc., all have to be assessed because these are the basics of health. If they are not in order, then the person's illness is likely caused by something other than a chronic condition.

It is very important to make sure you take care of the basics to build health, even if you cannot do everything at the beginning of your journey. One thing is better than none, two is better than one, and so on.

Creating Basic Health

Listed below are the parts and pieces of a healthy lifestyle. By taking the time to hone these skills, you are stepping powerfully forward toward the type of vitality, and therefore the health, you wish to have. One small shift toward health on a daily basis adds up over time to large changes and improvements.

Food

The primary function of eating is to stay alive. Non-human animals do not eat for pleasure or comfort; they eat because of a biological need. Their diets differ from one species to another. They are built to thrive on their ideal foods which vary from bacteria, plants, and other creatures. The diets of all these species have common elements. Their food is not processed; it is eaten in its whole and natural form. Their food has no added ingredients such as colors, flavors, or preservatives. Humans, on the other hand, eat not only for survival but for pleasure and comfort as well.

We have been designed to thrive on plants, fruits, nuts, seeds, fish, game meat, and grains, in their whole food form with little to no processing. Some foods must be processed, for instance, a food such as acorn flour is very nutritious, but it must have the tannins leached from it before it is used. The same is true with elderberries where the berries must be dried, frozen, or cooked before consumption. Both of those are examples of minimal, but needed, processing. The foods we were designed to thrive on supply fats, carbohydrates, proteins, and fiber along with vitamins, minerals, and other nutrients. Yet, the foods that commonly surround most people today are not always those which help them thrive.

Many of the foods widely available to people around the world create toxicity in the body because these foods are not in their whole form. Instead, they are ultra-processed with synthetic nutrients added back in to replace what is lost during processing. Additive colors and flavors must be used to make the food appealing because of processing, and preservatives and stabilizers are required to maintain shelf life and profitability. While there are certain vitamins and minerals added to processed foods, they are still missing enzymes, fibers, phytochemicals, and living organisms found in their non-processed and whole counterparts.

Much of the food on this planet has become a commodity of big business. When something like food is a commodity, it must be produced for the least amount of money in the greatest quantities possible to be sold at a price yielding the maximum profit. This has resulted in hundreds of thousands of easily available foods, many of which are nutrient-poor and toxic when consumed in large enough quantities.

What does all this mean? Humans are starving for nutrients. You might be wondering how this can be—I certainly think about it all the time. It turns out the relationship between humans and food is a long and complex story.

When it comes down to it, what you put in your mouth is vital to your overall health and well-being. Food fuels the body and provides important resources for it to heal. Most people have heard this at least once in their lives, but you literally "are what you eat". If your goal is to live your healthy enough life, proper diet and nutrition are essential.

Food provides three main building blocks called macronutrients. They are carbohydrates, fats, and proteins.

- Carbohydrates give cells and organs of the body instant and stored energy, aid in digestion by providing fiber, and form parts of DNA
- Fats help form the walls of cells and hormones, protect organs, and help keep the body warm in cold conditions
- Protein forms the structure of bones and muscles makes up receptors that allow cells to talk to each other, carries hormones and other signals through the blood, and maintain fluid balance in addition to other jobs

Additionally, certain foods provide micronutrients, known as vitamins and minerals, which the human body needs to function. Vitamins are made by living things (like plants and animals), while minerals are found in the earth. Some micronutrients are considered essential because the human body cannot make them; instead, they have to be consumed. Essential or not, the body uses these substances for thousands of functions. They are used to make energy to get through the day, maintain healthy muscles and bones, contribute to a strong and steady heartbeat, good circulation to detoxify unwanted substances, and for healing. These functions occur continuously, every day. If the body becomes deficient enough in a vitamin or mineral, symptoms of illness develop. For example, when Vitamin C is too low, a human can develop scurvy, a condition where the tissues can not heal and the immune system functions poorly. Vitamins and minerals are so important for human life that governments, doctors, and scientists all over the world keep track of and do research on them.

Food also provides us with fiber. Humans require fiber in their diet, in various forms in order to live a more healthy life. The Mayo Clinic reports,

> "Dietary fiber—found mainly in fruits, vegetables, whole grains and legumes—is probably best known for its ability to prevent or relieve constipation. But foods containing fiber can provide other health benefits as well, such as helping to maintain a healthy weight and lowering your risk of diabetes, heart disease and some types of cancer."

Almost no one, without making a specific effort to do so, gets enough fiber in their diet. Humans should be taking in between 20-40 grams of fiber a day, depending on the person and their age. Fiber can be found in soluble and insoluble types which are each important for different reasons.

- **Soluble** fiber comes from foods like beans, oats, peas, barley, apples, citrus fruits, carrots, and psyllium. It helps lower blood cholesterol and glucose levels.
- **Insoluble** fiber comes from whole-wheat flour, wheat bran, nuts, beans, and vegetables such as cauliflower, green beans, and potatoes. It promotes the movement of material through the GI system and increases stool bulk.

Table 1 includes some common fiber foods.

Table 1

Food	Serving size	Fiber (grams)
Beans	½ cup	5-9
Avocado	1 cup	9-11
Apple	1 medium	3-6
Artichoke	1 medium	6.2

Brown rice	1 cup	3.5
Pumpkin	½ cup	5
Potato	1 medium	5
Spinach	1/2	2.2

Sometimes, a certain food or foods trigger an inflammatory response in the body. For example, people with Celiac Disease cannot eat gluten. Gluten is a major part of many flours and an additive in lots of packaged foods. If those with Celiac Disease do not discover their gluten intolerance and eat foods containing it freely, they can become very ill and often develop chronic illness. Some people are sensitive to gluten even though they do not have as strong a reaction as those with Celiac.

People can be allergic or sensitive to almost any food and to any degree. A holistic doctor can assess sensitivities or allergies using a number of methods, tests, and elimination diets. The treatment is reducing or removing the foods, or other substances, that trigger an inflammatory reaction in the body and replacing the nutrition the problem foods provide with something else. A holistic dietitian or nutritionist, and many naturopathic doctors, can be particularly helpful with this part of the treatment by guiding you to alternatives that keep your nutritional intake balanced.

Other than modifications made for allergies or food sensitivities, the basic, overall healthy diet is one in which you:

- Eat a whole foods diet as much as possible (decrease/eliminate refined, packaged, and fast foods)
- Eat seven colorful fruits and/or vegetables each day
- Include fiber in your diet from vegetables and whole grains
- Eat plant fats primarily and animal fats sparingly
- Consume red meat sparingly and eat abundantly of fruits, grains, nuts, seeds, and veggies
- Eat a variety of food
- Limit sugar intake to occasional treats
- Decrease or eliminate all known food sensitivities/allergens
- Use a vitamin and mineral supplement as suggested by your practitioner

There are many resources out there if you want to learn more about the basics of food and nutrition including books, online courses, and local events. There are also many holistic doctors, dietitians, and nutritionists who can work with you to create a balanced and healthy diet for *you*. This is a sound investment in your overall health and well-being.

Soil Depletion of Vitamins and Minerals

The planet's soil has been degrading for years, and the vitamins and minerals in it are less than ever. This is a cause for concern because the body builds itself in part from the vitamins and minerals in the soil. When food is eaten, vitamins and minerals are extracted by the body so it can build and rebuild itself. The nutrients we eat fuel the millions of chemical reactions happening within our body at any given moment. If vitamins and minerals are not present in sufficient amounts in the soil, then they are also missing in the food we eat. As a result, it is not uncommon for a person eating all the fruits and veggies and living a healthy lifestyle to test deficient in a number of vitamins or minerals. This is why supplementing the diet with various vitamins and minerals is of the utmost importance.

Nutritional Supplements

Some people are able to get what they need *primarily* from food, while others must rely heavily on or choose to use packaged vitamins and minerals. Besides vitamins and minerals, there are a lot of other types of food supplements. Holistic practitioners use many different kinds of medicine from nature such as herbs (botanical medicine) and individual vitamins such as Vitamin C, minerals such as magnesium, essential fatty acids, and many more to assist the body with healing.

The quality of packaged supplements varies from one manufacturer to the next. A doctor of natural medicine will often prefer whole food-based products whenever possible to avoid unnecessary fillers and ingredients. The best clinical results are seen when folks use a multiple vitamin and mineral supplement, additional trace minerals, and whatever else their body needs to reach a healthy enough state.

What About "Organic"?

Organic can be defined as no chemical fertilizers, pesticides, or artificial agents, which includes genetically modified foods. Organic food products are premium items and command a premium price. Isn't it counterintuitive that clean, healthy, nutritious food without poisons is *more* expensive? But in today's societies, this has become a normal and accepted practice.

There is an incredible amount of information available today about organic foods. One very useful resource is the Environmental Working Group (ewg.org) which publishes a list of foods that should be purchased organically if you are able. If you enjoy learning, I would encourage you to read a few books and attend some free learning webinars about organic foods. Here is the bottom line: some foods should only be consumed if grown organically and some can be purchased non-organically. Keep in mind this is only taking into account the chemical effect on your body. Eating organic also reduces our impact on the planet.

Drink

Water is essential to life, and some cultures, such as Native Americans, hold water as sacred. The human body is made up of up to 60% water; even your bones are made up of roughly 31% water by volume. In general, to maintain hydration in the adult body, more than 32 ounces of water should be consumed daily. But keep in mind, this is really just a bare minimum. Water is needed to replace what is lost daily, about 1000-1200 ml, through the basic functions of urination, sweating and respiration. And water is needed for the millions of chemical reactions happening every minute of every day.

A common formula to calculate the average water intake for any age is ½ the body weight in pounds = ounces of water.

> **Example: A 100 pound person. 100 / 2 = 50. So, 50 ounces a day is a good place to start.**

If a person is super active, perspires, or feels thirsty, then they likely need more water. If someone eats a lot of whole, raw fruits and vegetables and is not very active they may need less.

Water is available through food but for the average person it is mainly supplied by the types of liquids drunk. Here are some tips:

- Consume plenty of fresh filtered water daily; depending on diet and exercise
- Quality is important; have your water tested if you are not certain about any impurities to see if you need a water filter

- Limit or eliminate caffeine consumption
- While some studies have shown one to two alcoholic beverages a day of a certain kind, like red wine, can have some health benefits, drinking more should be limited. Alcohol is a toxin to the body and even with minor health benefits, the net effect is that the body must detoxify the alcohol
- Decrease or eliminate soda and other sugary drinks; diet soda carries its own toxicities unless it is formulated with Stevia, a plant-based sweetener

Exercise

Exercise isn't just for weight loss. By moving your body, you increase blood circulation which carries oxygen and vitamins from your diet to every body system you have. In addition to improving brain health, it reduces your risk of cancer, heart disease, diabetes, osteoporosis, depression, and anxiety, among others. By exercising at least 150 minutes a week, research has shown the risk of dying from any cause decreases.

- Have a physical before starting any new exercise program
- Incorporate at least 30 minutes of regular exercise three to four times per week
- Find something fun to participate in, or enlist a family member or friend to get more motivation
- Learn a sport or activity that you can enjoy your whole life, like tennis, golf, cycling, or swimming
- Add cardio and resistance training as you are able, twice a week
- Walk everywhere you can, and take the stairs instead of the elevator, even if you walk the stairs for one or two floors to begin with; you can take the elevator the rest of the way
- Stretch every day
- Breathe deeply on a regular basis. You will have to train yourself to do this. An easy way to do this is to set an alarm on your phone for every 10 minutes. Stop and breathe deeply, fully expanding your chest. After a week, set the alarm for every 5 minutes; before you know it you will be breathing deeply on a regular basis

Sleep

Spending hours lying in bed may seem like a waste of time to some people when there is so much to get done. Realistically, this is very far from the truth. When sleeping, the body is able to repair and renew itself. Many adults in today's fast-paced culture find themselves sleep-deprived and at a higher risk for health issues like high blood pressure, obesity, type two diabetes, and mood problems like anxiety or depression. Keep in mind that your sleep will also improve as you work on other lifestyle habits, such as diet or exercise.

- Get 7-10 hours of sleep each evening; you know you are getting enough sleep when you feel rested in the morning
- Schedule time to prepare, relax and fall asleep and for stretching and waking up your body
- Stop evening activities (screentime) *at least* one hour before you need to be asleep
- Eliminate caffeine in the afternoon if you have difficulty sleeping

For more detailed information about sleep, see Chapter 18.

Mind-Body Connection

There is a clear connection between the health of the mind (emotions, self-image, support groups, dreams, aspirations, internal dialogue) and health. Part of this picture includes your stress levels. The more out-of-balance your thoughts are due to the pressure of work, relationships, family, etc., the more you should focus on supporting your mental health and well-being. The more positive and optimistic the outlook a person has, the healthier they are. The body stores past hurt and emotions as a physical memory, and this can make it difficult to heal the way we want to. Be patient with yourself. The following are all used to reduce stress.

- Stress relieving techniques, meditation, prayer, and journaling all have a powerful and healing effect on the body
- Walking in nature, especially in a forest, helps reduce stress and can be very grounding/balancing
- Making sure to spend some time with people who nourish your soul rather than those who bring you down

Environment

Decades of research have established that the environment in which humans live and work can impact their level of health. As science and society have developed, daily living and working spaces have become filled with more and more things that expose us to chemicals. There are a few steps you can take to help support your body's protective processes and reduce the effect chemical exposure has on your health.

- Use air and water filters; the cleaner your air and water, the less you impact your built-in detoxification systems
- Try to purchase thin-skinned fruits and vegetables as organic when possible to reduce your exposure to pesticides
- Avoid cooking and drinking out of plastic materials—choose glass or stainless steel instead to further reduce chemicals in your life
- Grow a plant or two in your indoor spaces; they can, depending on the species, help remove pollutants such as volatile organic compounds from the air
- Read labels! There are many ingredients in personal products, cleaning products, furniture, paints, flooring, and lawn supplies that can increase the body's toxic burden; the Environmental Working Group lists a number of ingredients to watch out for as well as a list of safer choices

Body pH

In general, the body must maintain a near-perfect pH balance. It is critical to the maintenance of good health. The symbol 'pH' is used to represent the acidity or alkalinity level. pH stands for 'potential for hydrogen'. Some call it the 'potential for health'. When checking alkalinity levels anything from 0-6.9 is acidic and from 7-14 is alkaline. The pH of the body varies, for example, in the blood the ideal pH is 7.35 to 7.45 which is fairly neutral, while in the stomach the ideal pH is 1.5 to 2.5, which is very acidic. Research and clinical medicine have established that smoking can create a lower pH, or in other words, a more acidic environment in the body.

Essentially every function of the body is dependent on the body maintaining a precisely balanced pH in the blood and other critical bodily systems. One of the key systems, for example, is the enzyme system. The enzyme system, as well as the electrical functions of the body, are dependent on electrolytes, essential minerals that are vital to many key functions in the body.

Electrolytes include sodium, potassium, chloride, bicarbonate, calcium, phosphate, magnesium, copper, zinc, iron, manganese, molybdenum, copper, and chromium. The most important for humans are sodium, potassium, chloride, bicarbonate, calcium, and phosphate.

Electrolyte levels are dependent on pH. This would indicate that without proper pH levels, it should be difficult for the cells to incorporate the necessary nutrients and energy for good health. This could lead to the cell weakening, which could lead to weakened tissue, and then to the organs themselves malfunctioning. This becomes even more serious as the body's systems are affected, leaving the body open to invaders of all types. It has been stated that poor health most often begins after the pH balance is impacted due to a deficiency of minerals, especially the electrolytes sodium, potassium, calcium, magnesium, and phosphorus.

Changes in pH do not have to be major: most elements of the body have a very definite pH range and slight changes impact chemical reactions both within and outside the cell. This is why the maintenance of pH levels is critical to overall body balance. To show the extreme opposites of the pH spectrum, a body that is too acidic may slip into a coma and a body that is too alkaline might slip into convulsions—neither is good. It is the proper balance that produces good health.

The bottom line when considering body pH for a smoker is to focus on those activities and strategies that create a more alkaline environment, counteracting the more acidic conditions established by smoking.

- **Common symptoms of pH imbalance include:** fatigue, mental fogginess, kidney and bladder stones, calcium and other mineral deposits, acne and other skin problems, insomnia, poor digestive function, low nutrient absorption, muscle pain and aches, joint pain and aches, osteoporosis, back pain, headaches and so much more
- **Things to avoid:** caffeine, all coffee, black tea, soda, sugar, processed foods, and a diet too high in animal protein
- **Things to include:** fruits, vegetables especially dark greens, whole grains, broth based soups, lemon water, complex carbs, herbal teas, balanced meals, essential fatty acids, and lots of deep breathing!

Detoxification

Your body has built-in systems that allow it to detoxify itself on a daily basis. Depending on how toxic your everyday environment is, your system can become overloaded and a therapeutic "detox" may be beneficial and needed. This is discussed in greater detail in Chapter 8.

Chapter 4:
A Tour of Natural Therapies

There are a number of different types of therapies used by practitioners of natural health. Many of these can be done at home, while others may need to be performed by a trained professional. This section serves as an introduction to each therapy and focuses on ways these therapies work to support health and recovery from illness. We will also take a look at things that have some research to indicate they may not be a good idea for a smoker. The Apothecary section contains more detailed information on how to use these particular therapies at home. It's important to realize whatever treatment, therapy, or substance is being used, the goal is always to support the body in its attempt to heal itself.

Botanical Medicine

Humans have co-evolved with plants in a mutually beneficial way and have protected and cultivated specific plants for millennia because humans have identified these plants as allies. Similarly, plants have shared their healing attributes with humans while using those same phytochemicals to heal themselves from harsh environments like flooding, heat waves, cold winters, or insect invasions.

Botanical medicine is the centuries-old method of using herbs and plants to heal. This is a practice used around the world, whether or not pharmaceutical agents are available. Humans consume herbs in many forms such as teas, tinctures, glycerites, salves, poultices, baths, essential oils, syrups, tablets, or capsules. Herbs can be used for babies, children, and adults of all ages. Many herbal formulas are available, and you'll read the discussion of them throughout this book. Here are descriptions of each so you know the differences between them:

- **Bath:** Herbal baths can include any combination of herbs; place herbs inside a muslin bag or cheesecloth and drop into a warm bath or hold them under a hot water stream
- **Capsules:** Powdered herb or herbs placed into a capsule and swallowed; these can be used for numerous health concerns
- **Essential oils:** Oil extracts from numerous plants are available for a variety of health concerns including physical immune

enhancement, emotional balancing, and physical and mental relaxation

- **Glycerite:** A liquid preparation of an herb made using vegetable glycerin to extract the medicinal constituents of the plant; it tastes sweet which makes it more palatable for children

- **Salve:** A semi-solid herbal preparation usually made with beeswax, olive oil (or some other type of carrier oil), dried herbs, and essential oils (if desired); salves are used topically for burns, wounds, rashes, boils, or other skin conditions

- **Syrup:** A viscous herbal preparation usually made with honey and varying herbs; it is used to soothe a sore throat

- **Tablets:** Single herbs or a combination of herbs blended together and either chewed or swallowed; these are generally used for people who don't like taking liquid or capsuled herbs

- **Tea:** Adding hot water to a dried herb, allowing it to steep for a few minutes, removing the herbs, and drinking it once it has cooled down; teas can be used for colds, coughs, relaxation, sleep problems, urinary complaints, and more

- **Tincture:** A liquid preparation of an herb through an alcohol or alcohol and water extraction process. It is usually made in a 1:5 ratio with one part of the herb being diluted in five parts of water. The dosage is measured in drops; they can be used for many conditions including coughs, colds, fevers, flus, or any time immune activation is desired.

- **Poultice and Compress:** A mass of plant material applied to the body and kept in place with a cloth; usually, made from fresh herbs—it will also work with dried forms

The commonly used botanicals for each system are listed in the corresponding chapter. The medicinal actions of the plants discussed in this book are often limited to the system being discussed. But, it is important for you to know that plants often have hundreds of actions on the body in various systems—many of which are beyond the scope of this book.

Homeopathy

The practice of homeopathic medicine, commonly called homeopathy, is over 200 years old and may be one of the safest and most effective therapies in existence. The medicines used in homeopathy are commonly referred to as remedies. These remedies are highly diluted substances that contain little to no molecules of the substance they are made from, but they do contain the information of the original substance. A homeopathic practitioner refers to these substances as potentized medicines. It is believed that when used correctly, the information carried by the potentized medicine assists the innate healing ability of the body, restoring balance and thereby allowing the symptoms of illness to resolve.

Remedies come in a variety of strengths. The common strengths available in most health food stores are 6C, 12C, and 30C. Other strengths, such as 200C and higher, are available online and from holistic practitioners such as Naturopathic and Homeopathic doctors. Remedies are affordable and easy to obtain. No prescription is needed and the typical cost is around $12.00 per tube. Each tube contains approximately 80 - 100 little white pellets to which a potentized medicine has been applied. A common dosing strategy is 3 pellets chewed or placed under the tongue, but the best dosing of a remedy can be very different from one person to the next. Dosing can also vary by practitioner, for example when using liquid dosing the dosing strategy would likely not be the same. Typically, in classical homeopathy a practitioner uses one remedy at a time, but there are some combination products commercially available that contain two or more potentized medicines.

The best way to dose these remedies is as needed, otherwise known in the medical world as PRN. Imagine you had a cough and started taking a remedy to relieve it. If the remedy you are taking is correct, the cough can be helped with a single dose. You will know when it is time to redose because the cough returns. At times, a remedy that was helping stops working. When that happens there are a few different changes the practitioner will make. They will either change the strength of the remedy or choose a different one. Most folks start with the strength of 30C, commonly available at the health food store. The next strength is 200C which usually has to be ordered from a practitioner or online. From 200C, the scale of strength goes to 1M, 10M, 50M. Many of the higher strengths (> 1M) must be purchased from a professional homeopath.

The success of homeopathy depends on how closely the symptoms you experience match the symptoms the remedy has been documented to produce. Remember, homeopathy uses the principle of "like cures like", meaning, if the substance can cause the symptoms in a healthy person then it can clear them in a person who is ill with those symptoms.

With homeopathic medicine, you want to take some time to discover the remedy that best describes *your* symptoms. If the remedy you choose does not describe your symptoms well enough, it will likely not work because you need a different remedy. A remedy more individualized to you and your symptoms. Discuss your needs with a professional homeopath who can prescribe a specific remedy that better matches your needs.

A homeopathic approach to healing can be very rewarding. When a correctly chosen remedy is used, it can work gently, efficiently, and without toxicity or side effects to relieve discomfort by assisting the body's healing. Homeopathic treatment is good for first aid, acute and chronic illness. Chronic care, often referred to as Constitutional, or Chronic Homeopathy, should only be done by a professionally trained homeopath and in some cases, one with formal medical training.

How to Use the Remedies for the Conditions in This Book

In some chapters, there are several possible homeopathic remedies discussed. It is important to note these are the most common remedies used, but they may not be the only remedies to consider. The remedies are listed by their full name followed by the common abbreviation in parentheses.

The symptoms any given remedy can be used to treat have been compiled into a vast collection of information called the *Homeopathic Materia Medica*. This book uses several different materia medicas and selected remedies that are specific to the symptoms discussed. It may be a little challenging at first to read the description of each remedy. But keep at it and you will get the hang of it in no time at all. Just keep in mind, in addition to these listed remedies being the most common, so too are the symptoms chosen. There may be other symptoms not listed.

Don't worry about choosing the wrong remedy! If the remedy you choose does not help, you can always try again. There is no mistaking a positive homeopathic response and once you see it, you will know what you are looking for. Helpful homeopathy books are listed in the Resource section of this book and suggested remedies are listed in the Apothecary section under Homeopathic Remedies.

Mind - Body Therapies

Research and clinical data have clearly established the link between a person's mind, how they think and feel, to their outlook and physical health. This is explored in great detail in the field of study called psychoneuroimmunology where questions such as, "Does how I think affect my health, really?" are asked and answered.

Mind-body therapies include meditation of all types, praying, breathing, biofeedback, neurofeedback, Neuro-Linguistic Programming, counseling, Qi Gong, Yoga, and many more. Throughout this book, there will be ideas and methods in which you can support your mind-body health. More specific therapies will be detailed in each chapter and in the Apothecary section.

Nutritional Therapy

As already discussed in Chapter 3, a proper diet is key to creating and restoring health. Creating the optimal nutritional status within the body before it becomes ill is the best strategy for managing one's health. Taking in food and drink provides the body with what it needs in order to mount an immune response and recover from illness more quickly. It supplies the nutrients a body constantly undergoing damage needs to heal and create new cells, tissues, organs, muscles, bones, nerves, and so much more. In addition to providing the basic nutrients, nutritional therapies are often used as a treatment. For example, a hot broth-based soup, rich in nutrients, can encourage the immune system to work better. Another great example is using fresh, colorful fruits and veggies to boost antioxidant status in the body. Someone not getting enough healthy fats in their diet might need supplemental essential fatty acids.

When thinking of nutrition as a therapy used to assist the body in healing, it helps to know the basic functions of the substances the body needs. The next section focuses on a few specific nutritional supplements frequently used for someone who smokes.

Frequently Used Nutritional Supplements

In addition to proteins, fats, carbs, fiber, vitamins, and minerals, some nutritional supplements are especially important for the smoking population which are detailed below.

B Vitamins

There are several B vitamins including: (Thiamin (B1), Riboflavin (B2), Niacin (B3), Pantothenic Acid (B5), Pyridoxine (B6), Biotin (B7), Folate (B9), Cobalamin (B12), Choline, and Inositol. B vitamins are water-soluble and are involved in several processes including methylation. Methylation is a biochemical process necessary for detoxification, and B vitamins are critical to this process. They also allow nerves to send and receive messages via electrical impulses. B vitamins help build and maintain the myelin sheath which protects nerves and allows for faster nerve impulses. They also help keep the inflammatory protein homocysteine in check. Homocysteine is a marker for cardiovascular disease risk and inflammation; this tends to be high in smokers. B vitamins are also necessary to make glutathione, and they help reduce genetic damage caused by air pollution.

You can take a B complex to supplement your diet with B vitamins, but caution should be exercised if you have kidney disease, as excess B vitamins are filtered by the kidneys. Some people report difficulty sleeping if B vitamins are taken too late in the day and riboflavin (B2) will cause the urine to turn bright yellow. Food sources of B vitamins include liver and other organ meats, beef, chicken, turkey, seafood like oysters and clams, legumes like lentils, black beans, pinto beans, eggs, leafy greens like spinach or romaine lettuce, and nutritional yeast. The amount of B vitamins each person needs varies depending on many factors such as lifestyle, diet, alcohol intake, volume of smoking, and stress levels.

CoQ10

Coenzyme Q10, otherwise known as CoQ10, is a lipid (fat) antioxidant involved primarily with energy production. It is present in almost all of your cells. The largest concentrations of CoQ10 are found in the most metabolically active cells such as the heart, liver, and kidneys. Without adequate levels of CoQ10, cells can't make enough ATP (the energy cells use to function), and this can lead to fatigue, weakness, low muscle tone, poor recovery from injury and illness, and a host of other symptoms. CoQ10 has been found to be protective against cardiovascular disease. As people age, levels of CoQ10 naturally decline, and although it is present in some food sources, eating alone doesn't seem to shift levels that much. It is also known that CoQ10 is lower in smokers, likely due to the increased need for CoQ10 due to the damage caused by smoking.

Clinical research suggests supplementation should be 100 mg - 200 mg of CoQ10 daily. As it is a lipid-based antioxidant, it is best absorbed when taken with food. You can also get additional amounts through your diet by adding CoQ10 rich foods. Examples include oily fish like salmon or sardines, organ meats such as liver or kidney, whole grains, spinach, cauliflower, broccoli, oranges, strawberries, or lentils.

Essential Fatty Acids (EFAs) & Fish Oil

As mentioned earlier, fats are one of the basic building blocks of nutrition, but not all fats are created equal. Lab tests look at the type of fat in your bloodstream, and that is one of the metrics doctors use to evaluate heart attack risk. Low-density lipoprotein (LDL) cholesterol is commonly referred to as bad cholesterol while high-density lipoprotein (HDL) is referred to as good cholesterol; the main difference is the size and hardness. LDL cholesterol is harder and will damage the arteries when there is too much in the bloodstream, while HDL cholesterol is more fluffy. Some LDL fat is important to maintain health, but too much is damaging to the blood vessels.

Essential fatty acids (EFAs) are one way to raise HDL levels while lowering LDL levels. These fatty acids come from both plant and animal foods. EFAs are the building blocks of cells' membranes, the structure which protects cells, gives them shape, and allows them to interact with the rest of the body. There are two broad groups of EFAs, omega-3 (alpha-linolenic) fatty acids, and omega-6 (linoleic) fatty acids. There are three main omega-3 fatty acids including alpha-linolenic acid (ALA), eicosapentaenoic acid (EPA), and docosahexaenoic acid (DHA). There are three main omega-6 fatty acids which are called linoleic acid (LA), gamma linoleic acid (GLA), and arachidonic acid (AA). Fish and animal foods contain EPA and DHA, while plant-based foods can contain ALA. EPA and DHA forms are easier for the body to utilize in comparison to ALA.

Both of these fatty acids, omega-3 and omega-6, are critical to good health. However, the human body does best when the ratio of omega-3 to omega-6 is 2:1. Many people get more omega-6 from their diet than is ideal, and this can create inflammation in the body. With modern diets, the omega-3 to -6 ratio is reported to be 1:16; this is much too high. In addition to a state of inflammation, this ratio puts a person at increased risk of many chronic diseases such as heart disease, diabetes, kidney disease, etc.

Omega-3s are anti-inflammatory, protective against cardiovascular disease, and have also been found to help with stress reduction. There are several ways in which you can add omega-3s to your diet. Fish oil is one of the easiest and it tends to be a cheaper option.

As far as supplements go, fish oil is one which you want to be particularly careful to make sure you are buying from a reputable brand. Look for a company that molecularly filters their fish oil; this ensures that you are getting a higher quality oil with no heavy metal concentrates.

Glutathione

Glutathione is very important to overall health and is the main antioxidant present in all cells of the body. It prevents damage caused by many different life exposures including smoking. When the body is ill, trying to detoxify, dealing with a lot of stress, etc., it needs and uses up more glutathione. The human body can make glutathione, but it needs three amino acids to do so: cysteine, glutamic acid (glutamate), and glycine. Of those three, the most important is cysteine. Boosting and replenishing glutathione happens when we have an adequate intake of protein from animal foods and plants. There is some good research that indicates taking a supplement called N-acetyl-cysteine (NAC) can help boost levels of glutathione in the body. This makes sense as NAC supplies cysteine, one of the most important molecules for glutathione. What is clear in humans is that the higher the levels of glutathione, the healthier the individual.

Multivitamins and Minerals

Multivitamins are critical given the state of the Earth's depleted soils and the poor diets of many humans. This is frequently part of nutritional therapy, especially when access to food is limited.

Usually, multivitamins contain some minerals, but barely cover the basics of what you need. There are over 4,000 minerals and only sixteen or so have been identified as important to health; these are what's included in a typical multivitamin. This is where supplements that contain trace minerals shine. Trace minerals supply a full spectrum of additional minerals in small amounts and clinically, people thrive with these extra nutrients.

Magnesium

Magnesium is a mineral that is responsible for over 300 chemical reactions in the human body. Some of these reactions include energy production, muscle contraction, protein structure such as in your bones, and optimal nerve function. Nutritionally it has been shown to help with diseases like high cholesterol, heart arrhythmias, metabolic syndrome, and even migraines. It is estimated that as many as two-thirds of western civilization does not have adequate amounts of magnesium in their diet. Cigarette smoking and alcohol consumption has been found to reduce magnesium levels in the blood.

Magnesium is becoming more deficient in the soil and food preparation, such as boiling, can also reduce the amount even further. Minerals such as magnesium require adequate stomach acid for optimal absorption. Taking it with a meal can increase your body's ability to absorb magnesium since there is more stomach acid being produced while you are eating.

The best sources of magnesium include green vegetables broccoli, spinach, chard, kale, legumes, cashews, sunflower seeds and other seeds, halibut, whole-wheat bread, and milk. Keep in mind, the standard American diet most likely won't supply adequate magnesium and some supplementation may be helpful for the vast majority of the population.

N-acetyl-cysteine (NAC)

NAC has been used as a medical treatment for disorders such as polycystic ovary syndrome (PCOS), preterm birth, acetaminophen (Tylenol®) toxicity, chronic bronchitis, ulcerative colitis, liver cancer, muscle performance, hemodialysis, asthma, Alzheimer's Disease, and Parkinson's Disease. It is an anti-inflammatory, antioxidant, and mucolytic (thins mucus to make it easier to cough up). New research in rats indicates it may be a promising agent to help reduce nicotine cravings; it seems to be the longer and more regular the dosing of NAC, the better the results, but more research is needed. Overall, research shows taking 600 mg of NAC once or twice a day is effective. The most common side effects included diarrhea, heartburn, and abdominal symptoms, although in general, NAC is well-tolerated at higher doses.

Probiotics

Probiotics are live microorganisms (in most cases, bacteria) that are similar to the beneficial microorganisms naturally found in your gastrointestinal (GI) tract. The most common probiotic bacteria come from two groups, lactobacillus and bifidobacterium, although many other types of bacteria are also classified as probiotics. Scientific evidence shows these probiotics:

- Boost the immune system by enhancing the production of antibodies
- Support the synthesis of vitamins and other nutrients
- Relieve the effects of, and treat, intestinal illness (diarrhea, constipation, IBS)
- Balance neurotransmitters affecting mood and mental state
- Prevent and treat vaginal yeast infections and urinary tract infections; and
- May reduce the risk of colon or bladder cancer

With 80% of your immune system located in your gut, having balanced intestinal flora is a major factor in defending your body against disease. Balanced GI flora is critical to the functioning of the immune system, the synthesis of nutrients, and detoxification. Balanced GI flora is also necessary for regular and normal bowel movements. Research shows there is a definite relationship between the gut, brain, and immune system.

Flora imbalances can be caused by poor diet, illness, use of antibiotics, and stress. Symptoms can include persistent gas, bloating, constipation, or diarrhea as well as anxiety, depression, and mood swings.

There are two ways to boost healthy GI flora: taking a probiotic supplement or adding probiotic-containing foods to your diet. Probiotic supplements come in liquid and capsule forms. Many of them are sold refrigerated. It is important to follow the storage instructions for your supplement—failure to do so could kill off the live, healthy bacteria it contains.

For centuries, if not millennia, humans have incorporated some sort of fermented food into their diet several times a week. Fermented foods provide a rich source of probiotic microorganisms beneficial to human health and include foods such as tempeh, natto, some cheeses, kombucha, miso and kimchi, and cultured dairy products such as yogurt and kefir. Be sure the food labels state "fermented" or, for dairy, "live and active bacterial cultures." When incorporating fermented foods into the diet, it is helpful to start with small amounts and increase serving size over time. This decreases the chance of gas and bloating which can happen when first adding fermented food to the diet.

Vitamin C

Vitamin C, also known as ascorbic acid, is an important antioxidant that has many functions in the body. It helps make collagen in the skin, tendons, ligaments, and blood vessels. Vitamin C is also critical to wound repair and forming scar tissue, helps repair and maintain teeth and bones, and even helps your body absorb iron from food more easily. It also plays a role in cardiovascular, respiratory, and reproductive organs. When you are severely deficient in vitamin C, scurvy can develop. Scurvy used to be common among sailors because they weren't able to access vitamin C-rich foods while at sea. The symptoms of scurvy include swollen and or easily bleeding gums, loss of teeth, fatigue and weakness, irritability, sadness, severe joint or leg pain, discolored spots (red, blue) on the skin, and easy bruising.

It cannot be emphasized enough that vitamin C is a potent antioxidant that helps the body cope with the free radical damage caused by smoking. Not having enough vitamin C, whether from food or a supplement, has been found to significantly raise the risk of developing COPD at a future date.

Vitamin C can be found in citrus fruits, peppers, strawberries, broccoli, brussel sprouts, or sweet potatoes to name a few. It is also available as capsules and liquid in varying strengths. Another option, besides supplementing with capsules, is to drink hawthorne or rose hip tea, both of which are high in vitamin C. Generally, the more you smoke the more vitamin C you use up. Most people can take high doses daily, but it can cause bowel upset and diarrhea if you choose to take a high dose orally.

Vitamin D

Generally, vitamin D is recommended for everyone who is living north of the 40th degree of latitude. In other words, it can be good for folks living north of the equator. During the winter months, there is not enough sunlight for the body to produce adequate amounts of vitamin D. This lack has far-reaching effects on the body. Vitamin D has been found to be integral to immune health, bone health, overall mood, and for an increased sense of well-being. It also has important anti-inflammatory effects. The ideal way to increase this vitamin in the body is to get out in the sun as much as possible. Food sources of vitamin D include fortified milk or margarine, fortified cereals, and fatty fish. Liquid forms of vitamin D are better absorbed than capsule-based ones and vitamin D is also more easily absorbed when taken with food because it is fat soluble.

Physical Medicine

Physical medicine includes a wide range of therapies used by practitioners such as naturopathic doctors, chiropractic doctors, acupuncturists, osteopathic doctors, and physical therapists. Some practitioners use physical medicine to restore proper structure to the body which then encourages optimal function within the body. Others employ physical medicine therapies to stimulate healing processes within the body. For example, lymphatic massage encourages the circulation of lymph, a clear fluid that circulates white blood cells and removes excess fluids in the body. Massage helps support immune function by moving metabolic by-products from the tissues into the lymph nodes where they can be neutralized. Other examples of physical medicine techniques that can be beneficial include skeletal and craniosacral realignment, muscle massage, dry skin brushing, and abdominal massage. Skeletal and craniosacral realignment work is often done by a chiropractic physician, naturopathic or osteopathic doctor, as well as other kinds of health practitioners with specialty training, such as massage and physical therapists.

Many physical medicine therapies such as dry skin brushing and abdominal massage can be done at home to help encourage health and healing. These therapies are discussed in the Apothecary chapter. Other therapies, such as muscle massage and skeletal realignment, are best done by someone with specialized training.

Topical and External Applications

Using topical and external applications is beneficial for much more than treating the skin. You may be familiar with applying a cream to a cut or scrape, but there is also powerful medicine to be found for the inner workings of the body through external applications. These types of therapies can include:

- **Compress (i.e. castor oil pack):** A cloth soaked in a solution, and like a poultice, is applied topically—designed to ease painful joints and muscles, draw out infection or deliver plant medicine through the skin; another word for compress is fomentation

- **Hydrotherapy applications:** As discussed in the next section, applications such as wet socks, heat or cold packs, contrast, heating wraps, and baths with natural medicine added to water

- **Liniment liquid or semi-liquid preparation (i.e. mint chest rub):** Used for delivering medicine, often essential oils or herbal medicine, through the skin

- **Poultice (e.g. onion poultice, mustard poultice):** A warm mass of herbs, or some other plant material applied topically that is designed to ease painful joints and muscles, draw out infection, or deliver plant medicine through the skin

In addition to soothing aching muscles and joints as well as delivering medicine, topical and external applications can also stimulate healing processes. They can encourage blood flow, relieve the body of heat, and help the body eliminate toxins and waste products. The Resources section contains a list of books and places to purchase these products.

Hydrotherapy

Hydrotherapy uses water as a method of healing. Although considered an old-world therapy, it is commonly used today in spas everywhere in the form of jacuzzis and steam rooms. A spa setting is meant for relaxation and stress release but when used therapeutically it is much more than simple relaxation. According to *Lectures on Naturopathic Hydrotherapy*, hydrotherapy can be used to stimulate immune function, increase blood circulation, and amplify natural detoxification. There are numerous forms of hydrotherapy treatments that you can do easily and safely at home as well as those that are usually administered by a naturopathic doctor or other natural health specialist in order to improve your overall well-being.

Constitutional Hydrotherapy

Constitutional hydrotherapy is a water-based therapy usually done by a professional. It causes superficial blood vessels in the skin to dilate and then contract. The contraction of superficial blood vessels brings blood into the internal organs, allowing them access to newly oxygenated blood, and increases the number of white blood cells.

In this therapy a person is wrapped up in a wool blanket, like a mummy, head uncovered. The blanket is opened momentarily so alternating hot and cold towels can be applied to the chest and upper back. Practitioners use a sine wave machine to gently provide electrical stimulation to organs that help with detoxification during therapy. The increased circulation brings more nutrients, oxygen, and white blood cells to all internal organs. It also allows the immune system to actively work while the body is resting, in fact, many people fall asleep or feel deeply relaxed after this treatment is completed.

Contrast Hydrotherapy

This therapy works through the placement of hot and cold towels over the chest and abdomen. When hot towels are placed on the body, superficial blood vessels dilate, bringing more blood to the surface of the body. When cold towels are applied to the chest and abdomen, the superficial blood vessels constrict, causing blood to rapidly flow into the internal organs. This action pumps more blood into the organs and directly acts on the thymus gland to increase the output of white blood cells. The towels should be placed in alternating succession, hot towels first and cold towels last, to promote this immune response. The secondary effect observed is a deep relaxation which helps the body naturally go into a repair state. The instructions for this at-home hydrotherapy are included in the Apothecary chapter.

Heating Compress

Heating compresses involve using cold water to stimulate the body's inner vitality by increasing circulation in the local area where the compress is. Additionally, because the heart and blood vessels are all connected in a closed system, the entire body is positively affected. Basically, a heating compress is taking a cold towel, thin cotton or flannel cloth, and placing it on an area of the body. The body will send more blood to the area in an attempt to warm up the towel (this is where the term "heating compress" comes from). Blood carries more nutrients and oxygen in and more wastes out of the affected tissues which evokes a healing response in the area.

Soaking Baths

These baths can be used to relax, heat up, or cool down the human body as well as support a healing response. Essential oils of lavender or chamomile can be placed in the bath to help support calmness throughout the body—a few drops is plenty. A bath with herbs (oats, lavender, comfrey, or calendula) can be soothing to the skin and relaxing to the nervous system.

Caution: It's important not to place a person with a fever in a cold bath because the change in temperature can shock the body, potentially starting a seizure. Additionally, essential oils aren't for everyone either as they can aggravate some people's skin.

Steam Inhalations

This therapy involves breathing steam from warm water with or without essential oils added. Essential oils are suggested because of the immune-stimulating effects they have. One to two drops of essential oils are sufficient. Steam inhalations are generally used by people who have upper respiratory conditions like stuffy noses or congested sinuses.

Wet Socks

Wet socks are considered to be a type of hydrotherapy; this treatment involves wearing well-wrung-out wet socks covered with a thick pair of dry socks and allowing the body to dry them out. Typically done overnight, this therapy can stimulate the immune system, drain congestion from the head and chest, relax away aches, increase circulation, and aid in detoxification. The exact process is outlined in the Apothecary section if you want to try this one at home.

Supplements to be aware of...

Just as some plants in nature can be poisonous, some nutrients and other natural therapies can also be harmful. Therapies heavily depend on what disease process is going on in the body. Concerning smoking, there are a couple of things you should be aware of.

Beta Carotene

Beta carotene is a pigment in plants that creates the vibrant yellow, orange, and red colors of some fruits and vegetables. It is a provitamin A; this means an enzyme is needed to react with beta carotene and create a form of vitamin A the body can use. It is a potent antioxidant that can help with skin health, improve vision, and in general, is protective against some types of cancer.

Since the 1990s, scientists have known the risk of lung cancer in active tobacco smokers taking high-dose beta carotene is higher than that of non-smokers and former smokers. This means smokers should not take high-dose beta carotene found in beta carotene products, vision-supporting supplements, and certain multivitamins. A prospective study of French women found the higher the dose of beta carotene, the higher the risk of lung cancer in smokers. The risk remained even at a lower dose of an estimated 2.1 mg daily. At this point, more research on this subject is needed. Please consult with your doctor before starting any supplements with beta carotene if you currently smoke.

Alpha-tocopherol

There has been some discussion over the years that alpha-tocopherol, the most common supplemental form of Vitamin E, supplementation is dangerous in tobacco smokers. At the time of this publication, there is not a lot of research indicating Vitamin E supplementation is harmful to smokers. One study from 2008 indicated use of alpha-tocopherol supplementation in smokers who smoked over five cigarettes a day and were either in the lowest or highest weight categories had a 14% increased risk of developing pneumonia as well as an increase in tuberculosis risk.

Other research supports alpha-tocopherol supplementation. One study followed thousands of male participants over thirty years looking at all-cause mortality. The men who had higher amounts of alpha-tocopherol in their blood had a 17%-47% lower mortality rate depending on their age and health habits. This was seen even among men who smoked and/ or consumed alcohol. Another Vitamin E study looked at male Finnish smokers from ages 50-69 who also were getting 90 mg of Vitamin C or more in their diet on a daily basis. In men ages 50 to 62, there was an estimated increase in mortality by 19%, but those who were ages 66-69 had a 41% decreased risk of mortality.

All antioxidant vitamins tend to be decreased in every smoker due to the oxidative nature of cigarettes. If you'd like to supplement with Vitamin E, a mixed tocopherol Vitamin E is recommended, as this is closer to how it occurs in nature. Alpha-tocopherols tend to be synthetic in many cases, and this may be what contributed to the negative opinions on Vitamin E supplementation in smokers originally. This area needs further research.

You can create health through what you do every day from the choices you make. This includes your use of natural medicines. Remember health is a journey, and it can take time to get where you want to go. Humans can find change incredibly hard, especially in the beginning. By putting one foot in front of the other and focusing on your goals, you can get there.

Chapter 5:
A Tour of the Smoker's Body

The human body is nothing short of a miracle. It seems to have been designed to withstand an onslaught of environmental, biological, and mental attacks. Humans breathe in polluted air, eat and drink toxins, and observe and experience trauma *every day!* Yet, even with all that, most people continue to find health and even thrive in what many call a hostile world.

The human body has the propensity to be as healthy as it can be at any given moment. This means humans can self-heal, as can most organisms on the planet. A simple example is when you get a cut. Your body's built-in healing systems get to work straight away, and you don't have to do anything besides keep the wound clean.

There are times when healing happens very slowly. Other times it happens not at all. Many different things influence self-healing such as the overall state of health, the frequency of damage (is it a one-time thing or ongoing), and the severity of the damage. Is it the first drink of contaminated water or the thousandth?

Let's say you are really healthy and once in a while, you have a smoke. Your body can repair the damage from that one instance quickly with little to no lasting damage. Make no mistake here—even smoking one time creates damage in the human body. But as soon as the smoking stops, the body starts to repair that damage. Cells designed to remove toxic substances will flood your lungs, mouth, blood vessels, and other organs to start cleaning up the toxins deposited. Oxygen levels that fell during smoking will rebound. Carbon dioxide levels that increased during smoking will start to normalize. Poisoned cells will be removed, recycled, and replaced by other cells.

If, on the other hand, you are a person who smokes multiple times each day the picture is different. The body does not typically heal that quickly and while you continue to smoke, the body can not heal from the damage. However, there are ways to mitigate the damage and support the parts of the body that are being injured each time you have a smoke. The best option is to stop smoking altogether as soon as possible, but saying someone needs to quit is much easier than actually doing it. If this is not an option, then the next best thing is reducing the damage smoking causes. This is made possible because the speed at which a body heals or dies can be influenced.

What Happens in the Smoker's Body?

First, let's take a minute to understand what is taking place in a smoker's body every time they smoke and what the cumulative damage is from ongoing smoking. Subsequent chapters go into greater depth system by system, including how you can support each system, but until then here is a quick look at what is happening.

There are about 600 chemicals in the average cigarette. When a person lights the tobacco on fire, they inhale 7,000 chemicals in addition to nicotine. There has been sufficient research conducted to know two things. One, smoking harms most organs and cells in the body. Two, there are at least 70 known cancer-causing chemicals present in tobacco smoke. Some of those chemicals are:

- **carbon monoxide:** a colorless, odorless poisonous gas—in large doses, this chemical can cause death quickly because it takes the place of oxygen in the blood. In smaller doses, such as in people who smoke, it makes it harder for oxygen to get to their organs and muscles.
- **metals:** including arsenic, beryllium, cadmium, chromium, cobalt, lead, and nickel
- **oxidizing chemicals:** highly reactive chemicals that can damage the heart muscles and blood vessels
- **radioactive compounds:** polonium-210 and lead-210 are both cancer causing
- **tar:** solid particles suspended in tobacco smoke

These chemicals affect many parts of the body including the respiratory, cardiovascular, reproductive, and immune systems. They also have a detrimental effect on the skin, muscles, bones, nerves, metabolism, and brain.

Every single time a person smokes, they can experience:

- Irritation of the trachea (windpipe) and larynx (voice box)
- Swelling and narrowing of the lung airways
- Excess mucus in the lung passages
- Reduced lung function
- Impairment of the lungs' clearance system

- Damage to the air sacs of the lungs
- Increased blood pressure
- Increased heart rate
- Constriction of blood vessels in the skin
- Decreased blood oxygen
- Blood that becomes more prone to clotting
- Damage to the lining of the arteries
- Reduced blood flow to extremities (fingers and toes)
- Increased risk of stroke and heart attack
- Drop in immune function
- Decreased antioxidants in the blood
- Tightening of certain muscles
- Increased risk of stroke and heart attack
- Eleven-minute loss of life

With repeated smoking over a relatively short time, certainly over an extended time, smokers can exhibit all of the above plus:

- Increased risk of bronchitis, pneumonia, influenza, and lung cancer
- More severe and longer-lasting illnesses in general
- Reduced bone density
- Lower sperm count
- A higher percentage of deformed sperm
- Genetic damage to sperm
- Impotence
- Reduced fertility
- Menstrual cycle irregularities
- Early menopause
- Increased risk of cervical cancer
- Greatly increased risk of stroke and heart attack
- Irritation and inflammation of the stomach and intestines
- Increased risk of painful ulcers along the digestive tract

- Reduced ability to smell and taste
- Premature wrinkling of the skin
- Higher risk of blindness

Additionally, a person who smokes throughout their life is at higher risk of developing a range of diseases, including:

- Cancer: lung, mouth, nose, larynx, tongue, nasal sinus, esophagus, throat, pancreas, bone marrow (myeloid leukemia), kidney, cervix, ovary, ureter, liver, bladder, bowel and stomach
- Lung disease: chronic bronchitis, COPD, bronchiolitis, and emphysema
- Atherosclerosis
- Ulcerative conditions of the digestive system
- Osteopenia, osteoporosis, and bone fractures
- Type 2 diabetes
- Rheumatoid arthritis
- Gum disease (periodontitis)

Some Eye-Opening Statistics

Humans are very good at counting how many people do certain things so they can make financial projections. Let's take a look at some statistics used in the tobacco industry to track those who use their products.

How many worldwide tobacco smokers are there?

As of July 2021, the World Health Organization estimates there are 1.3 billion smokers on the planet. Over 80% of these are people in low- and middle-income countries, and in general there are more male smokers than females. The number of smokers in the world dropped about 6% from 2005 to 2021, though roughly 14% of the world continues to smoke.

What age are people starting to smoke?

Most adults report that they started smoking in adolescence, typically in their high school years. Not to mention, children of smokers are more likely to start smoking than those of non-smokers.

How successful are people who try to quit smoking?

According to most major health agencies around the world, only 8% of people are successful in their attempt to quit smoking for at least 6-12 months. If you are among the other 92%, don't lose hope. This book is designed to help you find your healthiest self while you continue your fight for nicotine independence.

What is the tobacco industry worth?

Tobacco is a lucrative business. In 2020, the worldwide tobacco industry was estimated to be worth 760 billion U.S. dollars. By 2025, the value of the worldwide tobacco market is expected to exceed 888 billion U.S. dollars. Turns out, killing people slowly results in huge financial returns.

What is the cost of smoking?

The cost of a pack of cigarettes has steadily increased over the years. For Americans, the cost has gone from 25 cents per pack in the 1950s to 8 dollars a pack in 2022. In nearly all countries, tobacco is also heavily taxed. Not only do smokers have to worry about the accumulated financial burden of smoking, but should realize the steep cost to their life. Table 2 is a breakdown of what smoking will cost your life over time.

Table 2

One cigarette	11 min
Pack of 20 cigarettes	3 hours 40 min
Carton of 200 cigarettes	1.5 days

While this information seems bleak, don't be discouraged. There is much you can do to support your body.

The Body Heals

The human body is always healing itself. When the body is in the process of healing, there are often symptoms. Symptoms such as inflammation, discharges, pain, fatigue, fever, and overall weakness to name a few. Sometimes these symptoms can be detected or felt in the body, and sometimes the symptoms are so mild they aren't even noticed. When a system in the body is overburdened with things that need to be healed, it is not uncommon to see a lot of symptoms, including more severe ones. When the body is supported in its attempts to heal, healing happens quickly.

How quickly does the body start to heal once smoking stops?

If you pair quitting with actively trying to help your body heal, the results can be almost unbelievable! Look at what happens after you stop smoking for certain time periods as displayed in Table 3.

Table 3

20 Minutes	Pulse and blood pressure start to drop, closer to normal; hands and feet warm-up
8 Hours	The amount of nicotine and carbon monoxide in your blood drops by 50%
12 Hours	Carbon monoxide level normalizes
24 Hours	The risk for heart attack because of smoking starts to drop
48 Hours	Senses of taste and smell get sharper as your nerve endings start to heal; lungs kick out mucus and other gunk left from cigarettes; you don't have any more nicotine in your body
30 Days	Breathe easier, have more energy, lungs start to recover and will keep getting better
2 Weeks - 3 Months	Lungs are stronger and clearer, your blood flow has improved, you can exercise without getting as winded, and your risk of a heart attack goes down even more
3-9 Months	Deeper, clearer breaths, instead of hacking, you cough in a helpful way that actually clears things out, fewer colds and other illnesses, increased energy
1 Year	The risk of heart disease is now half of what it was a year ago
5 Years	Chances of a stroke and cervical cancer are now the same as a non-smoker, half as likely to get cancer of the mouth, throat, esophagus, or bladder
10 Years	Compared to someone who still smokes, you're now half as likely to die from lung cancer and the chances you'll get cancer of the larynx (voice box) and pancreas both drop
15 Years	Chances that you'll get heart disease are the same as if you never smoked, your body has done a ton of recovery and healing

Remember your body is always trying to heal itself. Some things it can take care of quickly and easily, while other things can take years. The less damage being done to your body, the more healing it is capable of doing.

As you read through the coming chapters try to not become overwhelmed. It is a lot of information. Read each chapter to get a more complete understanding of how everything fits together. You can always revisit what doesn't make sense the first time and in *A Smoker's Daily Plan*, everything is condensed into practical and applicable steps.

Chapter 6:
The Air We Breathe

The only reason life, as humans experience it, is able to exist on Earth is because of the unique mixture of gasses in the atmosphere. At sea level, the air is made up of about 78% nitrogen, 21% oxygen, and up to 5% of water vapor in some areas of the planet. Various other gasses including argon, carbon dioxide, neon, helium, and other trace gasses make up the last 1%.

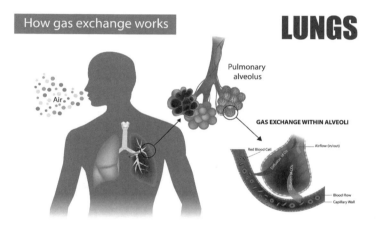

Every day, to stay alive, humans need to breathe oxygen from the air and get rid of poisonous by-product gasses like carbon dioxide. This is called gas exchange, when the lungs take in oxygen and get rid of carbon dioxide. The exchange happens within the alveoli of the lungs, a part of the respiratory system which also includes the nose, mouth, throat, voice box, and windpipe. This collection of body parts works together, collaboratively with other systems in the body, to allow us to breathe and live. Sometimes a respiratory system stops working as it should, and treatments such as oxygen, respirator, surgery, etc., are used to artificially preserve life.

The Respiratory System

The lungs are the main focus of the respiratory system. They are basically tubes (bronchial tubes) and sacs (main lung) that are able to take the oxygen in the air and attach it to red blood cells. The oxygen is then carried by the red blood cells through the rest of the body. When the body uses oxygen it produces carbon dioxide (CO_2) which is then sent back to the lungs to be breathed out. This system also includes the nose, mouth, throat, voice box, and windpipe that serve as the conduit for air to move in and out of the lungs.

Human lungs work like the handle on a manual well pump. When the handle goes up, the lungs expand via the diaphragm muscle and take in oxygen, and when the handle goes down, the lungs collapse and push out CO_2—the waste from the cells. The lungs are made of dense, spongy tissue filled with tiny air sacs called alveoli; this is where the gas exchange happens. The alveoli are rich with very small blood vessels called capillaries that bring CO_2-rich blood into the lungs—they can release it and then pick up oxygen to carry to the rest of the body.

When air is breathed in through the nose and mouth, it travels down larger bronchi into smaller and smaller tubes until it gets to the alveoli. It is easiest to imagine the bronchus (plural of bronchi) as an upside-down tree with smaller and smaller branches or pipes that air can flow through. The bronchus, and nose, are lined by cilia which are finger-like projections coated in mucus that captures dust, pollen, and other particles. Cilia in the bronchial system move rhythmically to help move particles up and out when you inhale things; these particles are what stimulate the cough reflex to clear debris from the lungs.

How Smoking Affects the Respiratory System

Once you put flame to a cigarette toxins are released. Cigarette smoke contains thousands of chemicals including gasses, particles, and dangerous free radicals. Free radicals are excited bits of energy that will bounce around and damage the body if left unchecked. Luckily, humans have several antioxidant mechanisms to deal with this, but smoking in any amount can overwhelm these systems depending on a person's overall health.

For example, a substance present in smoke called acrolein is toxic to cilia, tiny hair-like structures in the lungs. Since cilia are what help move debris out of the lungs, any particles you inhale sit in your lungs rather than being coughed up. Smoke also impairs lung defenses and has been linked to increased asthma and other non-cancerous lung disorders. Formaldehyde, another substance present in cigarette smoke, is also toxic to cilia and irritates the lungs. Cadmium, arsenic, and lead can all be found in cigarette smoke as well; these heavy metals are dangerous to humans. Cadmium specifically can promote emphysema, one of many chronic lung diseases.

Emphysema is one of several diseases of the lungs, including chronic bronchitis, classified as Chronic Obstructive Pulmonary Disease, or COPD for short. These diseases are generally more common in smokers but can happen in non-smokers. The main factors in calculating COPD risk are breathing in cigarette or pipe smoke, air pollution, fine particles, and chemicals.

How to Support the Respiratory System

What's most important to keep in mind is how the body is always attempting to heal itself. The lungs have incredible ways of dealing with chemicals, toxic gasses, and particles from the external environment, including smoking; therefore, the most important step in restoring a smoker's body to health is for them to stop smoking. Often it is not the first step. Keep this in mind as you read about other possible ways to support your body.

This is a great time to review Chapters 2-4 if you have any questions. These chapters contain the basics of health that are often referred to throughout the rest of this book.

Supplements

N-Acetylcysteine (NAC)

A study conducted in rats showed that in addition to supplying cysteine for glutathione, N-Acetylcysteine may also help with lung fibrosis. Fibrosis is damaged connective tissue in the lung. In this particular study, NAC reduced the thickness in the tubes, increased the size of the air sacs, and decreased inflammation.

In the case of people with COPD, NAC has been found to reduce the number of exacerbations although it does not seem to improve lung function. The best results were found with people taking NAC regularly for over six months. Thus far, it doesn't seem to matter if low doses or high doses are used as both are effective at reducing the severity of exacerbations or attacks. These attacks include symptoms like shortness of breath, cough, and sputum production. For more information about NAC, see Chapters 4, 8, and 9.

Glutathione

When it comes to the respiratory system, researchers have found time and again decreased levels of glutathione present in people with various respiratory conditions including asthma, COPD, acute respiratory distress syndrome (ARDS), idiopathic pulmonary fibrosis (IPF), and cystic fibrosis (CF). Smoking introduces damage to the lung tissue directly and without supplementation; many smokers have chronically low and depleted levels of glutathione. For more information about glutathione see Chapters 4, 8, 10, and 18.

Vitamin C

Smokers who smoke one or more packs per day are at a high risk of "severe hypovitaminosis C". In other words, smokers have such a decreased level of Vitamin C in their body that their health is at risk. People who smoke less than a pack a day are at a reduced risk, though their Vitamin C status can still be lower than optimal. For more information about Vitamin C, see Chapters 4, 7-9, 11, and 18-20.

Botanical

Thousands of years of oral and written history show that people and plants have a rich and complex history. Plants are food and medicine for the human body. There are many plants on the planet with an affinity for the tissue of the respiratory system. Some of these particular herbs are listed here and act in different ways, but they are all considered potent respiratory system medicine.

Mullein

Mullein (*Verbascum thapsus*) is a plant that has antioxidant, antiviral, anti-inflammatory, and antispasmodic qualities. Traditionally, it has been used most often for respiratory complaints including hoarseness, tonsillitis, cough, asthma, and bronchitis. It is most commonly used as a tea infusion or boiled into recipes in the kitchen. This particular herb is great because it helps prevent coughs, and when you do cough, it makes the cough more productive to help clear the gunk out of your system. It is also soothing due to its mucilaginous quality; mucilaginous plants can be very soothing to different tissues in the body.

Lungwort

Lungwort (*Pulmonaria officinalis*) is traditionally used in many countries to support the lungs and help with conditions like pneumonia, asthma, chronic bronchitis, laryngitis, or cold and coughs. It can help reduce the occurrence of coughs, make coughs more productive, and can help increase sweating. Sweating can be useful when your body is trying to overcome illness because it helps flush toxins from the body.

Due to its high phenol content it is a potent antioxidant, though it appears to be quite safe. Evidence demonstrates it is a moderate anti-inflammatory herb; research has also shown lungwort works on pathways partly responsible for chronic health diseases including cardiovascular disease. If you decide to use this herb, you can take it as a tea. See the Apothecary chapter for more details.

Schisandra

The berries of schisandra (*Schisandra chinensis*) are traditionally used in Chinese medicine to help with cough and asthma due to their antioxidant and anti-inflammatory effects. It is also liver-protective and has shown the ability to help regulate the immune system. In animal models, it was shown to reduce damage in lung tissue caused by smoke exposure in comparison to subjects with no smoke exposure.

Smoking, over time, can cause chronic lung inflammation depending on how much and how often someone smokes. Schisandra can help reduce that chronic inflammation. If you decide to try this herb, research shows the most effective way to take schisandra for cough is in an alcohol base such as in a tincture.

Nettle

Urticaria dioica, more commonly referred to as stinging nettle, is a stinging plant that grows in almost every state in the United States. Traditionally and through modern research, it has been found to be an anti-inflammatory, antioxidant, supports faster wound healing, helps maintain healthy blood pressure, and is supportive of the urinary system. It also provides minerals including iron, Vitamin C, carotenoids, and even fatty acids which are very important in smokers. A smoker's body uses up more vitamins and minerals to maintain health because of the poor air quality due to smoking. Nettle also seems to help with allergic rhinitis which can be caused by, or worsened by, smoking according to some studies.

Through an herbalist or other trusted resource, you can educate yourself on what the plant looks like. From there you can harvest it yourself, but be aware! Stinging nettle isn't called stinging for no reason. Gloves are recommended if you adventure into the forest to harvest this yourself. You can also purchase loose-leaf nettle from any reputable herb company instead.

Be sure to know what type of nettle you need as there are three different parts of the plant which can be used including the leaf, root, and seed. The root supports urinary health, the leaf is an antioxidant and anti-inflammatory with a mild diuretic action, and the seed is considered an adaptogen that supports the adrenal glands and the body's overall response to stress. For more information about nettle, see Chapter 9.

Gotu Kola

Centella asiatica, commonly known as gotu kola, is considered the "elixir of life" in Chinese culture. It has many different actions including anti-inflammatory, antioxidant, and antiviral. It assists with wound healing, is liver protective, and even helps protect the nervous system. Gotu kola has also been found to have anti-cancer properties for several cancers, including lung cancer.

This herb has been used traditionally for lung health to help support connective tissue which becomes damaged from smoking over time. Gotu kola has been shown to support thicker skin when wounds are healing; it can also make the tensile strength of the healed wounds stronger according to research. For more information about gotu kola, see Chapters 11 and 15.

Calendula Mouthwash and Gargle

Calendula officinalis flowers have healing properties for skin and mucosal tissue—tissue that lines the inside of organs like the GI tract and openings of the body, such as the mouth and nose, and which often secretes mucus. The trick is, the oils from this plant work best when they come in contact with the surface of the tissue. For example, when a person smokes, they damage the tissues in the mouth. A calendula mouthwash allows the herb to wash across the inner surface of the mouth and can stimulate healthy tissue and heal the damage. For more information about calendula, see Chapters 11 and 16.

Lifestyle

Of course, the basics always apply when it comes to lifestyle. This might be a good time to revisit Chapters 3 and 4, as they are important to understanding the basics of creating good health. Included here are some extra and more in-depth things to consider.

Diet

With the lungs specifically in mind, there are a few nutrients that may help. First, it is important to remember antioxidants. Antioxidants work to decrease the damage caused by living everyday life. Oxygen itself, which humans require to live, is damaging because it is a free radical or oxidant. Eating more antioxidant-rich fruits and vegetables can help prevent this damage. Smoking causes more damage due to oxidation and having at least 4-5 servings of fruits and vegetables a day helps with this. Dark berries such as blueberries, blackberries, or boysenberries are loaded with antioxidants because of substances called anthocyanidins. One study evaluated the reduction of lung function over ten years, and found vegetables such as tomatoes and carrots can help protect the lungs from damage due to poor air quality.

Secondly, a mineral called selenium is a potent antioxidant. It isn't as common in dietary foods because of modern farming practices. Selenium increases the body's primary antioxidant system by increasing glutathione activity in the lungs. This can reduce the growth of lung cells which may help reduce lung cancer, one of the most deadly cancers in the United States. Selenium can be found in foods such as tuna, turkey, chicken, salmon, brazil nuts, seeds: sunflower, chia, and flax, whole grain breakfast cereals, and various sun-exposed mushrooms.

One last thing to note, relative to lung capacity and lifestyle choices is the involvement of alcohol. Research shows alcohol generally reduces lung capacity in smokers, but wine consumption, in moderation, may reduce lung damage due to its antioxidant activity.

While diet is discussed in numerous chapters of this book, an in-depth discussion can be found in Chapters 3 and 4.

Breathing Exercises

Breathing exercises can help improve how well you can move air in and out of your lungs, especially if you have already been diagnosed with COPD.

Lungs have a built-in recoil which means your muscles don't always have to do all the work. As you exhale, the weight of your chest and the elastic quality of the lung tissues helps push the air out.

When you have a chronic lung disease, this elastic quality of the lungs is decreased as well as the CO_2-oxygen air exchange. Over time, the diaphragm isn't able to work as effectively at drawing in fresh air. This compounds the problem.

There are two well-researched techniques that show positive benefits. You can do one or both of these on a daily basis.

Pursed Lip Breathing

This type of breathing will help you relax and breathe better by releasing air trapped in your lungs. It can also help you catch your breath more easily if you find yourself huffing and puffing from exercise or other daily activities like lifting or walking up stairs. Begin by closing your mouth and breathing through your nose to a count of two. This should be an easy breath with the

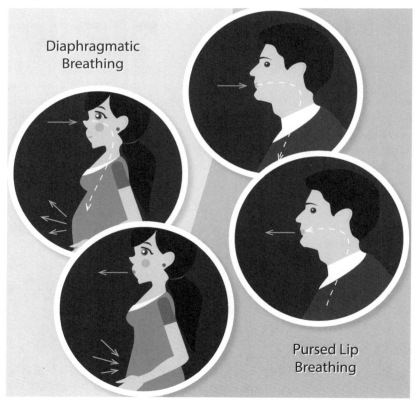

muscles in your upper body as relaxed as possible. Next, double the amount of time you exhale (count of four) through puckered or pursed lips. This exercise should be done in a relaxed state focusing on breathing out longer than you breathe in. Initially, this should be done more often during the day (around 4-5 times or so) until you start feeling results, then you can reduce this to 2-3 times a day daily.

Belly Or Diaphragmatic Breathing

The goal of this breathing exercise is to help strengthen the diaphragm muscle which will help you breathe easier. This particular exercise may be easiest to try lying down rather than sitting up until you get used to it. You can put pillows under your head and your knees to make yourself more comfortable. With one hand on your upper chest and one hand on your abdomen, breath in slowly through your nose and then exhale slowly through pursed lips. When you exhale, your upper chest should move as little as possible. Once you have this down, you can start practicing this exercise in a seated position, but only if that works well for you. You can do this 3 or more times daily for 5-10 minutes at a time.

Other Therapies to Consider

Acupuncture

Having a hard time breathing is a common symptom after years of smoking, especially during exercise or other intense physical activity. Acupuncture has been shown to help improve breathlessness in more severe cases of chronic disease including cases of COPD. With at least two weeks of treatment, all studies included in the analysis showed acupuncture made breathing and exercising easier.

Steam Inhalation

Steam inhalation is easy to do at home and requires very little equipment. First, boil some water in a pot on the stove. Once it has reached boiling, remove the pot from the stove and pour the water into a glass or ceramic bowl. Lean over the bowl and place a towel over your head to trap the steam. Concentrate on breathing slowly and deeply to allow the steam to reach deep into your lungs. The therapy time varies as it depends on how long the steam lasts. Steam inhalation is more effective when you add 2-3 drops of essential oil to the water in the bowl.

There are several different choices of oils which you can try. One study found that lavender essential oil has the potential to reduce lung inflammation and help support your immune system. Another oil to consider would be tea tree oil if you suspect you have any sort of lung congestion. Please keep in mind that essential oils are very concentrated essences from plants and some essential oils can be dangerous. Always do your research and consult a health professional before using a new essential oil.

Lymphatic Massage

The lymphatic system assists the body in removing toxins that accumulate over time. This can be especially helpful for smokers as they accumulate an increased load of toxins daily. A lymphatic massage can help move the lymph through the body and is best done just before showering along with dry skin brushing.

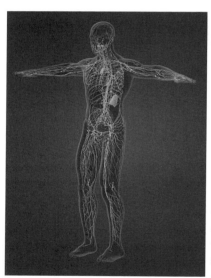

Lymphatic drainage massage was developed in Germany to treat lymph-edema, a condition involving fluid accumulation, most often seen in post-mastectomy patients. However, modern quality of air, water, food, and other elements can cause a significant build-up of metabolic waste products even in an otherwise healthy body. This includes toxins from smoking which can result in low energy, fatigue, and mood swings. Lymphatic massage can help by increasing the volume of lymph flow by as much as twenty times, vastly increasing the system's ability to remove toxins and infectious materials. If you are generally healthy, the do-it-yourself version of this technique may help you shake off fatigue and cold.

More information about this can be found in the Apothecary section.

Homeopathy

The homeopathic approach, as briefly mentioned in Chapter 3, is designed to select a potentized remedy that most closely matches a person's individualized set of symptoms. But much like potentized arnica can help the majority of bruising injuries, so too are there remedies that have been found helpful for a smoker's cough. These will not cure anything, especially while you are still smoking, but they can often help relieve symptoms in a non-toxic way.

The following set is a good pool of commonly selected medicines for smoker's cough. They also present the more common variations of how this cough is experienced by smokers.

- **Bryonia:** Best used for a dry and painful cough, with a dry throat, and intense thirst, it is often worse after eating or drinking. There may be a frequent desire to take a long breath to expand the lungs. Sometimes there is a feeling as if the chest would "fly to pieces". Frequently there is a tough mucus in the trachea, loosened only with much coughing. The cough may be triggered when entering a warm room and/or by speaking. The pain is often relieved by staying immobile or applying strong pressure to the ribcage. If the person is coughing while lying down, they must sit up to get relief.
- **Caladium:** A cough, with difficulty in raising mucus, is the highlighting symptom for this remedy; it might be the only symptom. The cough is usually relieved once the mucus comes out. Additionally, there may be a feeling of constriction in the larynx and trachea which makes it difficult to breathe deeply. The cough may be sudden and involuntary, triggered by a tickling high up in the throat (above the larynx).
- **Drosera:** A remedy commonly used for a dry or barking cough that is worse at night and from the warmth of the bed. It can be triggered by speaking or laughing, with a feeling of tickling in the throat or crawling in the larynx. There can be a feeling as if there is a feather or piece of dust tickling the throat. There may be fits of uncontrollable coughing, sometimes so bad that the person ends up vomiting. The hard coughing may cause the person to become hoarse or even lose their voice. The cough may sound like a whooping cough. It is generally worse towards evening and after midnight, in a warm room or with warm drinks, and typically gets better in the open air.
- **Hepar sulphuricum:** This is a remedy for a cough that can appear in different forms, such as dry and hoarse, but the most common symptom found in a smoker, is a loose or rattling type of cough. There may be a sense of suffocation or wheezing and breathing difficulty along with the cough. The mucus may be yellow and/or

blood-stained. It tends to be worse from dry cold winds, cool air, cool drinks or food, the slightest draft, when any part of the body gets cold or uncovered, being touched, lying on the painful side (if there is one), and in the morning. It's better in damp weather, from wrapping the head up, from warmth, and after eating.

- **Lobelia inflat**a: This cough is often accompanied by a sense of chest constriction and a feeling of suffocation. Painful and labored breathing is often present. There may be a sensation of heaviness or a feeling of weight in the chest. Nausea and vomiting are frequently present with the cough, but not always. Coughing is worse after smoking, in the afternoon, from movement, and when cold—especially cold washing. Better by rapid walking, toward evening, and from warmth.

- **Nux vomica:** The cough covered by this remedy often comes with oppressed breathing (difficulty getting a full breath, tightness in chest while breathing) which is frequently, but not always, experienced at night. The cough may be dry or rattling and may have bloody mucus. The cough is often dry, hacking, and teasing and can appear as long coughing spells that create stomach pain, vomiting, and may make the person's head ache. The person is likely impatient, irritable, oversensitive to sound, light, smells, and cold drafts. In general, they are often chilly and like to be wrapped up in a blanket. The cough is worse from both mental and physical exertion, at night, and in the morning. The cough may be better in warm open air (loosens up) but may be worse in cold open air. There can also be an improvement from sipping warm drinks.

Chapter 7:
The Blood Running Through Our Veins

Imagine a stream high in the mountains during summer. The water, coming from the last bits of melting snow, bubbles and babbles down the cracked stones, tripping its way around rocks and roots as it skips gently down the slope. All along the way, thirsty plants like pine trees, grasses, and mosses are getting a drink. Animals are also coming to the stream hunting for food and sipping sweet cool water. Now, imagine how full of life this water has to be to sustain this ecosystem. It must be clean of contaminants and rich in minerals. It must also have a thriving culture of microbiotic life to sustain itself. The mountain stream is what provides life to this environment.

Like a mountain stream, your circulatory system is linked to every tissue in your body and is made up of the heart and blood vessels. Imagine your red blood cells rushing through your blood vessels, spinning quickly through every twist and turn, delivering fresh oxygen and nutrients to the body along the way. Red blood cells also pick up wastes and carbon dioxide as they travel, speeding off to deliver those products to organs like the liver or lungs for elimination. Delivering all substances required for life is what blood does, and it is the primary way the body is able to keep itself alive.

Consider what happens if your blood is too thick or lacks minerals. It wouldn't be able to carry as much oxygen as you need or pick up enough carbon dioxide. When the composition of the blood is poor and the vessels carrying this precious substance are damaged, the risk for many different illnesses is high. Sadly, due to lifestyle choices and habits, environmental toxicity, and modern society, this story of poor blood composition and damaged vessels is surprisingly common in today's society. This is especially true for the smoker. The good news is that there are many things you can do to support your body and improve the composition of your blood and lymph.

The Cardiovascular System

The cardiovascular system is made up of the heart and the blood vessels. First and most important, is the heart, an organ essential to life. You can live without a gallbladder or a spleen, but if your heart stops beating, permanent brain damage can occur within minutes, and death follows a few minutes after that without rescue intervention.

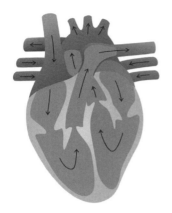

The heart is made up of four chambers, two smaller atria which are located in the uppermost portion of the heart, and two larger, more muscular ventricles below the atria. When blood enters the heart, it does so through the right atria which pushes blood into the right ventricle. The right ventricle sends blood rushing into the lungs where it drops off carbon dioxide and picks up oxygen. Blood then heads back into the left atria of the heart and into the left ventricle, the most powerful chamber of the heart. The left ventricle is responsible for pushing blood throughout the rest of the body. The heart itself has its own pacemaker, but your brain signals the heart to beat as needed to support blood flow for whatever activities you are doing. If you are hustling up a flight of stairs or sprinting after a running toddler, your heart is beating much faster than if you are sitting in a forest contemplating the beauty of nature.

As for the blood vessels, they are more than just passive pipes blood rushes through. There are two types of blood vessels: arteries and veins. Arteries contain oxygenated blood from the heart and lungs, and they also have muscular walls to help blood move along. These look pink or red under your skin, and they are more round. Veins contain deoxygenated blood which can look blue in appearance. These vessels have very little muscle mass; so, they are flat beneath the skin. The pumping of blood through the body, breathing, and the body's muscles contracting as we move, all help the veins get the blood back to the heart, so it can move to the lungs and release toxic carbon dioxide.

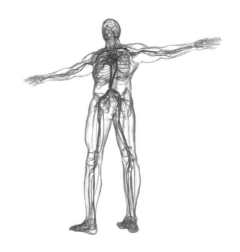

As previously discussed, blood is critical to life as it carries nutrients and oxygen to all cells, as well as carries out wastes and carbon dioxide. This means the heart and lungs work in conjunction as an oxygen source and pump sending blood out. This interaction has an effect on every organ and system in your body, which is why supporting your heart and lung health is so important.

How Smoking Damages the Cardiovascular System

It has been estimated that smoking doubles the risk of developing heart disease. As heart disease is one of the most common causes of death worldwide, this relationship between smoking and heart health can't be ignored. According to the Surgeon General's report in 2014, congestive heart disease, stroke, aortic aneurysm, and peripheral vascular disease are linked to smoking. Smokers have been shown to have worsening heart disease risk factors over time, one of the more common being a narrowing in arteries due to increasing carotid artery thickness. It comes down to this, smoking damages the blood vessels.

Cigarette smoke generates free electrons or reactive oxygen species which causes injury and inflammation to the inside of the blood vessels. Inflammation is your body's way of dealing with any sort of injury or infection. This is part of how you heal yourself. It's also important to keep in mind that the smaller the vessels, the more at risk of damage those vessels are. This is particularly important when you consider the coronary arteries around the heart. When those start getting blocked, it can cause angina, an intense squeezing chest pain. As a side note, nitroglycerin, a therapy for angina, has been shown to be less effective in smokers.

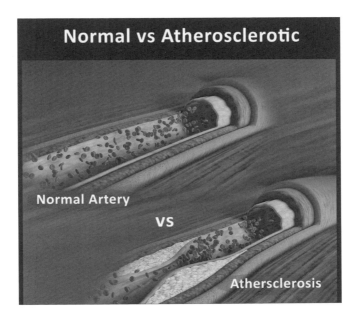

Once injury to the blood vessels has happened, there is a greater risk of atherosclerosis.

This simply means the walls of the arteries are being fattened up by cholesterol depositing inside the vessel to serve as a bandaid for the injury. Over time, this narrows the diameter of the artery and reduces blood flow which can lead to heart attacks, strokes, and impotence in men depending on the vessel affected.

How to Support and Heal the System

Now for some good news: when a smoker lights up fewer times, the risk of developing cardiovascular disease also goes down. The main focus in supporting the cardiovascular system is to help protect the structural integrity and surface of the blood vessels. This is possible through a variety of natural options.

Many of the options listed to help support the health system have been introduced in Chapters 2-4. Please refer to them for additional information, as they are the basis of information used throughout this book. For example, the following common supplements are introduced in great detail in Chapter 3.

Supplements

Vitamin C

In addition to its antioxidant properties, vitamin C is important for rebuilding and protecting body tissues. Blood vessels get damaged over time and vitamin C can help stimulate the endothelial cells to multiply in addition to increasing collagen production. These are the cells that line the inside of all of your blood vessels. Vitamin C also helps prevent cellular destruction and helps preserve nitric oxide, an important vasodilator that helps maintain a healthy vascular system. For more information about Vitamin C, see Chapters 3-4, 6, 8-9, 11, and 18-19.

Fish Oil

Essential fatty acids (EFAs) are important to the overall health of almost every human on the planet, but they are especially critical for smokers. Fish oil is a good source of fat for the body because fish concentrate the omega-3s naturally available in algae. We in turn take advantage of these omega-3s when we consume fish. EFAs specifically help modulate stress hormones, are anti-inflammatory, and help reduce cardiovascular disease risks. For more information about EFAs, see Chapters 4, 9-10, 14-15, 17, and 19.

Magnesium

Research has shown magnesium can lower blood pressure by a few systolic and diastolic points when adequate amounts are taken over a span of roughly one to three months. When taken regularly for four or more weeks in heavy smokers, it has also been found to reduce the number of cigarettes consumed in a day. Magnesium has also been found to lower the risk of sudden cardiac events by up to 77% in women.

It's important to keep in mind that the standard American diet most likely won't supply adequate minerals for you, so some mineral supplementation is helpful for the vast majority of the American population. 500-1,000 mg of magnesium daily has been shown to positively impact the cardiovascular system and overall well-being in many people. For more information about magnesium, see Chapters 4, 8, 15, and 18.

Botanicals

Dark Berry Extracts

Dark berry extracts are highly condensed preparations of fruits like blueberry, blackberry, elderberry, etc., which are rich in bioflavonoids. Bioflavonoids are polyphenolic compounds that have been shown to support strong cell growth and deliver an anti-carcinogenic effect. This is important for a body already at increased risk of abnormal cell growth and certain cancers due to daily smoke exposure.

Current research also suggests that bioflavonoids may help promote cardiovascular health, as well as potentially offer protection from neurodegenerative diseases such as Parkinson's disease and Alzheimer's disease. A relatively high intake of flavonoid-rich foods and beverages has also been suggested to improve processes that take place within the blood vessels (vascular endothelial) for a short period of time.

Turmeric

Turmeric (*Curcuma longa*) has been used for generations in India for many different diseases. The rhizome (similar to a plant root) is the part used medicinally, and it has been shown to have many positive health effects, many of which can be helpful to smokers. Turmeric is anti-inflammatory, antioxidant, antimicrobial, and has many anticancer mechanisms. It can even lower cholesterol, making it protective to the entire cardiovascular system.

Hawthorn

Hawthorn (*Crataegus spp.*) has been used in herbal medicine around the world for centuries including in Europe and China. It is well-known as a cardiac tonic, but it has also been used for gastrointestinal complaints, gallbladder disease, and respiratory illnesses like shortness of breath and asthma. It is a potent antioxidant, anti-inflammatory, and has anticoagulant properties.

It can also help increase the force of the heart's contractions and can dilate narrowed blood vessels which is helpful in diseases like congestive heart failure. It has shown the ability to protect the heart in cases of ischemia/reperfusion injuries which is especially important in folks who are at risk of having a heart attack or stroke. Ischemia/reperfusion refers to the sudden return of blood flow to tissue that was lacking it. This can also cause injury. Hawthorn, specifically the berries, has lipid-lowering effects that are protective for small blood vessels. Research has shown hawthorn is protective of mitochondria in the heart. Mitochondria are responsible for energy production in almost all cells in the body, but their highest concentrations are found in heart muscle.

Lifestyle

The foundations of health including diet, water intake, sleep, and exercise can't be emphasized enough in relation to the heart and blood vessels. The effects of the heart touch every single cell in the body; therefore, it makes sense that everything you do on a daily basis can impact your cardiovascular system in some way. Of course, the basics always apply when it comes to lifestyle. You may wish to revisit Chapters 3 and 4 before continuing. Included here are some extra, and more in-depth, things to consider when working on ways to better your health.

Diet

- Beetroot

    Adding beets (*Beta vulgaris*) to your diet is a great way to improve your overall health, especially if you smoke. This vegetable can increase nitric oxide which dilates the blood vessels and allows greater blood flow. Beetroot juice can increase oxygenation in muscles as well as lower platelet aggregation which reduces the risk of blood clots. It can also lower blood pressure. Beets are loaded with antioxidants which are protective of capillaries and other small blood vessels making them a great addition to any diet.

Beets are easy to find at your local grocery store throughout the year. Keep in mind foods high in nitrate can put an additional burden on your kidneys. This is well-tolerated by healthy folks, but be sure to consult with a health professional if you have any kidney problems before adding beets to your diet.

Once you know if beets are right for you, they are easy to incorporate into a lot of recipes. One way to enjoy them is to dice up some fresh beets with sweet potatoes and sauté them in coconut oil, or whatever healthy oil you have on hand, for about 15 minutes or so. Sprinkle cinnamon over the top while they cook. Add diced-up beet greens, cover for 3-5 minutes, then serve.

- Chromium

    Chromium is an essential mineral that is naturally present in the soil and is required in *trace amounts* for optimal human health. Insulin resistance occurs when cells are unable to use insulin, causing glucose to build up in the blood, leading to damaged blood vessels and various organs over time. Chromium has been shown to lower insulin resistance by helping cells use insulin and glucose better. Research supports this, proving it can be helpful in diabetics, especially since chromium is low in that population.

    Chromium picolinate is the most easily absorbed form of chromium. A daily dose to help maintain blood sugar health is at least 200 mcg a day. Chromium can also be found in foods such as egg yolks, whole-grain foods, nuts, green beans, broccoli, meat, and brewer's yeast. For more information about chromium, see Chapters 4 and 13.

    Note: There are other forms of chromium that can be toxic to humans; these are being investigated through scientific research all over the planet.

- Salt and Potassium

    Salt intake, otherwise known as sodium chloride, should be reduced to 2.3 grams (roughly 1 teaspoon) a day. Sodium is critical to good health, but when it is consumed in excess, disease can set in. In countries where salt isn't used as much in foods, blood pressure tends to be in a normal range as a person ages. Sodium intake directly correlates to high blood pressure. Research shows within weeks of lowering dietary salt intake, blood pressure drops to a more normal level. This means the more salt you eat, the more likely you will have high blood pressure, especially as you age.

    Potassium is a mineral prominent in vegetables and helps lower high blood pressure. improving your sodium-potassium ratio does more for you than just lowering your sodium intake alone. Newer research suggests as you work to lower your salt intake, you should also work on raising your potassium levels. This can be done with a more whole-foods-based diet. Potassium-rich foods include dried fruits (raisins, apricots), beans, lentils, potatoes, winter squash (acorn, butternut), spinach, broccoli, leafy greens (beet, chard, kale), avocado, and bananas.

    Sodium is a common preservative in the modern food industry, because of this it's important to keep in mind eating fewer processed foods can be even more important than reducing how much salt you cook with at home. The vast majority of Americans eat processed foods which are probably part of the reason heart disease mortality is so high in America. Processed foods are commonly high in sodium and low in potassium. As you work on implementing change, remember that processed food includes food from the grocery store, as well as fast food, and other restaurants.

    Overall, the key here is to use salt in moderation and eat more vegetables, just as your parents should have told you as a child. Sodium and potassium are both needed to maintain a healthy nervous system, hormone balance, and immune system. Using a little salt to flavor your whole food meals is perfectly fine and even encouraged. Remember, moderation and knowing what you are consuming are key.

Other basic dietary recommendations include eating plenty of vegetables and dark berries. Both are chock full of nutrients that help protect the blood vessels from further damage and help them to heal.

Exercise

Exercise has been shown through thousands of studies to have a positive effect on the body regarding many diseases, especially in relation to heart disease. Living a sedentary lifestyle with little physical activity is a leading contributor to poor heart health—this is true despite other risk factors such as smoking, high blood pressure, or high cholesterol. Exercise has been shown to improve cholesterol levels by raising HDL cholesterol, and lowering LDL cholesterol and triglycerides which are markers for cardiovascular disease risk. Blood pressure can be lowered and the heart strengthened through exercise.

If you've been living a sedentary lifestyle, even if it has been years, it is possible to turn your heart health around. Studies have found the risk of death and heart disease has been lowered or reversed in men and women who start up an exercise routine. This includes those who are middle-aged. Be sure to consult your doctor before beginning any exercise routine, especially if you haven't exercised in a long time. It's best to start with something small like walking 15-30 minutes a day, joining a yoga class, or even checking out qigong. It is a gentle exercise used in China for centuries as part of their general healthcare system. In many countries, Qigong is such a natural part of life that people will gather for a quick session on the side of the road. Any person passing by can join if they wish but there is no obligation to do so.

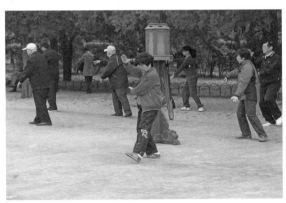

More information about exercise can be found in Chapter 3.

Other Therapies to Consider

HeartMath®

HeartMath® is a collection of techniques, research, and technology that brings together years of research on the connection between the heart and brain. HeartMath® was developed as a way to help people maintain more control over their blood pressure and heart rate variability (HRV). HRV refers to how the heart is able to regulate your blood pressure up and down depending on the activities or thoughts you are having. It is also an important factor in how resilient to stress you are. This can change from one heartbeat to the next.

Research has found the heart beats more erratically during stressful situations and with negative thoughts and emotions. This impacts how well the brain works, limiting higher functions that impact problem-solving and decision-making skills. This may be a big reason why people don't always make the best decisions under duress. Similarly, maintaining a positive mental state works the opposite, meaning your brain works better when you are relaxed. If you are able to keep a more positive outlook and emotional state, the heart's rhythm is more even and balanced.

If you are interested in trying this technique for yourself, HeartMath® offers a free 90-minute video where you can learn more about it and how it may improve your overall health and well-being (at the time of publishing). You can also find qualified practitioners who can walk you through their system step-by-step. Learn more about HeartMath® at www.heartmath.com.

RESPeRATE™

The RESPeRATE™ is an FDA-approved non-medical device which helps you breathe better. The device works by guiding you through an exercise designed to slow and deepen your breathing. Slowing down your breathing also slows down your heart rate, and can help promote relaxation which allows for increased blood flow. RESPeRATE™ is most successful when used regularly for approximately 15 minutes a day. Some people have even been able to use this device to lower their blood pressure medication dose. This device is now available for purchase online. Learn more at www.resperate.com.

Chapter 8:
Our Internal Detoxification

The modern world is full of toxins in many different forms. The air we breathe, the water we drink, and the very soil we use to grow food are subject to chemicals developed or isolated in a laboratory somewhere. Some of these toxins were developed with a benign purpose in mind such as protecting plants against pesticides, or creating more durable plastics, while others such as tear gas were created with a more malicious intent.

The U.S. Environmental Protection Agency (EPA) has classified over 185 air pollutants as hazardous. This includes gasses like benzene or asbestos and elements from the periodic table like mercury or cadmium. Toxins exist in your home from flooring, paint, and the furniture you sit and sleep on every day. Even fragrances from personal care products count as chemicals. Air pollutants can cause several different types of cancer, damage your nervous system, cause fertility difficulties and birth defects, eye and nasal irritation, coughing, wheezing, and most especially, cardiovascular damage. Damage occurs over time with each exposure, be it large or small.

There are naturally occurring elements in the soil that can be dangerous as well, but in most cases, they aren't concentrated enough to cause harm to humans. Nature in general is supposed to be a safe place, but whether from natural disasters, human activities like mining, or accidents such as spills and leaking underground tanks, the soil can be contaminated. The EPA monitors the majority of these sites, though the number is constantly changing as new sites are added and old sites are cleaned up. The dust from contaminated sites can carry toxins a long way to expose humans and wildlife, and contaminated soils can cause water pollution.

Water is necessary to life, and because of this, it's important to make sure the quality and purity of your water is the best you can afford to get. Water treatment, when using a public water system, cleans out many contaminants but the process itself uses some chemicals which may leave harmful byproducts. Microbes from fecal wastes can pollute water despite water treatment, and some groundwater is contaminated by nature including deposits of heavy metals or radioactive isotopes. Agriculture and other industrial businesses can leave chemicals like pesticides, solvents, heavy metals, or even petroleum products in water as well. This includes lakes, streams, and aquifers. Exposure to these chemicals can cause a myriad of short-term and long-term side effects including organ damage, fertility issues, and nervous system damage among others.

Finally, you should realize your home probably has toxic by-products to which you are exposed to on a daily basis. Research looking at common household dust found forty-five different chemicals present, most of which qualified as being endocrine disruptors. This means the chemicals in your household dust can cause problems in your reproductive and hormone-signaling systems. Some more common household chemicals include phthalates, perfluorinated chemicals (PFCs), and flame retardants.

Air filters, water filters, plants in your home or office, etc., can help get rid of these chemicals from your environment before your body is exposed to them. But, what if you can't afford those filters? What if you aren't able to buy green furniture due to the often, much higher expense? Is all hope lost? Your body is equipped to deal with toxins, even in today's heavily contaminated world. Remember the purpose of this information is not to scare or overly worry you, but rather to help you understand exactly how many chemicals are in the daily environment. Your body has systems in place to deal with these toxins in small to potentially moderate exposures via the detoxification system. Of course, this system can be overwhelmed, especially with large or chronic exposures such as smoking. Thankfully, the body has a way to detoxify itself.

The Detoxification System

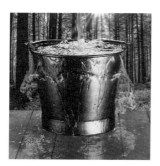

The most important concept of this chapter is to understand what detoxification is. On a basic level, it means removing toxins from the body. Today, "detoxification" is a word commonly used in the alternative health community. Once people understand how much they are exposed to chemicals on a daily basis, this concept of cleaning out the toxicity from your body makes more sense.

Now, think of a metal bucket—brilliant silver, shining in sunlight. This bucket represents you and your toxic load. When you do restorative activities such as eating lots of vegetables, exercising for at least 30 minutes a day most days of the week, laughing with friends, etc., the toxin level in the bucket goes down. When you eat junk food, stay up too late streaming movies or watching cat videos, yell at your partner for whatever reason, spend your day sitting in front of a computer, smoking, etc., the bucket fills up. Symptoms occur when the toxin level overfills the bucket. This means your detoxification systems are not keeping up with the workload. Skin rashes, joint pain, headaches, fatigue, gastrointestinal complaints, and insomnia are just a few examples of symptoms that can arise and manifest differently for each person once they have exceeded their tolerated toxin load.

Your detoxification system is a complex interworking of different organ systems in your body. The main organ of this system is the liver, but all detox organs are required to keep the body healthy. This list also includes your skin, lungs, kidneys, lymphatics, and gastrointestinal tract (especially the bowels). Your entire body works to optimize your built-in detoxification. Vital nutrients and oxygen are carried by your blood into those organs, and the waste is removed. These are the organs that help get rid of waste so your body can work as efficiently as possible.

Liver

The liver is one of the most amazing organs in the human body. It's tucked up on the right side of your abdomen where most of it is protected by your ribcage.

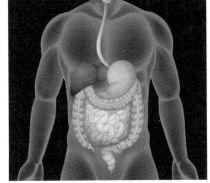

Despite weighing only three pounds on average, it has over 500 functions that have been discovered thus far. It helps with digestion by producing many things including bile to process fat and carry wastes, making proteins and factors for the blood for transporting fats and hormones, making cholesterol, and storing excess blood sugar as glycogen (stored energy for future use). The liver also regulates amino acids and clotting factors in the blood, converts toxic ammonia to be excreted in the urine, processes hemoglobin and bilirubin (byproducts of red blood cell breakdown), eliminates drugs and other poisons, and even supports the immune system by filtering the blood and making immune factors. The liver is also a storage place for vitamins and minerals.

Kidneys

The kidneys are located near the back wall of your chest cavity just above your lower ribs. They are normally about the size of your fist, and they are one of the hardest-working organs in your body. Kidneys work to control fluid balance and drinking plenty of water helps support your kidney health, so they can do their work more efficiently. Kidneys help control the pH level (acid-base balance) of your blood and electrolyte balance. They also play an important role in maintaining proper blood pressure, producing a hormone that signals red blood cell production, activating Vitamin D so your body can use it, and helping get rid of toxins and wastes. The kidneys and liver work together to do the majority of the filtering action required to maintain good health.

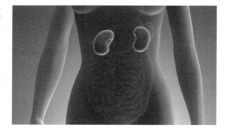

Gastrointestinal Tract

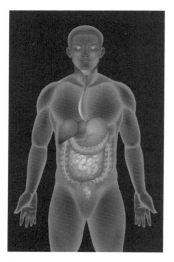

The gastrointestinal tract (GI tract) is an important member of the detoxification team. The foods eaten, unless grown at home without chemicals, are exposed to pesticides and other substances as they travel the food chain from farm to local supermarket. When the GI tract is functioning as it should, the body is good at absorbing the nutrients it needs, and leaving behind what it doesn't. The GI tract is also home to millions upon millions of bacteria which, among many things, also produce substances the body needs to detoxify. For more information about the GI Tract, see Chapter 16.

Lungs

The lungs are an important part of the body's detoxification system, especially in smokers who are constantly exposed to toxins and chemicals. The body excretes waste products (CO_2 and particulate matter) through the lungs an average of 850 times each hour, 20,200 times each day, and 8,103,000 times each year. That translates to around 650,000,000 toxic expulsions over a typical lifespan. This important function is one way the body maintains pH balance and eliminates many different substances. Breathing is an ongoing, automatic process and a valuable activity for detoxification. For more information about the lungs, see Chapter 6.

Skin

The skin is the largest organ of the body and is covered in more detail in Chapter 11. The skin is part of the body's detoxification system due to its sweating ability, this will be covered in greater detail in the therapy section. Please keep in mind there are some medical professionals out there who discount the skin's ability to support detoxification since the liver and kidneys do the bulk of the work, and a quick internet search will reveal these dissenting opinions. For naturopathic and other natural medicine doctors, sweating is an important way to rid the body of toxins and tonify several body systems.

Lymphatic System

Not least important is detoxification through the lymphatic system. This system, with over 500 filtration and collection points, circulates lymph fluid which carries away metabolic wastes, bacteria, viral agents, and poisons. Lymph flow is encouraged by exercise, deep breathing, and regular body movement. Toxins can be stored within lymph nodes for a long time but eventually become too toxic for the body to manage.

It's important to remember that all the parts of the body work together in concert. It's easy to compartmentalize each organ and its function, but these are just pieces of the whole health puzzle. It is impossible to disregard the body and how it integrates. The blood carries nutrients in and wastes out to other organs to be filtered. The nervous system oversees all of these activities and helps adjust body functions as needed to help optimize the detoxification process.

How Smoking Affects the Detoxification System

After understanding what the detoxification system is and how it works, it becomes clear how smoking burdens this system. In addition to everyday detoxification from food, stress, and the environment, it's possible to see what a profoundly negative impact smoking can have on these organs and the system in general.

By smoking every day, you are adding to your body's daily toxin burden. As it takes time for the detoxification systems to eliminate toxins, this burden builds up. When your body can't keep up anymore, symptoms develop such as cough, fatigue, muscle and joint pain, headache, slow healing, and so much more. This is also part of the reason why smokers are more likely to have fatty liver disease, cancer, heart disease, stroke, diabetes, and lung diseases like emphysema or chronic bronchitis.

How to Support and Heal the Detoxification System

Whether you are still actively smoking or recently quit, there are ways you can help support your detoxification systems. Detoxification is a steady process that can require time depending on your years of chronic toxin exposure and the fullness of your bucket. It is crucial you are eliminating wastes via your bowels, kidneys, lymph, and sweat. But, if you push too hard on these systems, you may feel ill from the detoxification process. Signs of pushing the detox systems too hard are headaches, fatigue, skin rashes, and GI upset. Keeping that in mind, it is important to make sure you reach out to a health professional to help support and guide you through detoxification.

There are many nutrients, minerals, and vitamins your body must have on hand for the chemical reactions needed to properly detoxify. Many people jump right into a cleanse without understanding how a massive dump of toxins from the body can make one feel really ill and in some cases, create more damage. Remember to be gentle with yourself, easy does it. Begin your detox by taking small steps, for example, if you don't drink adequate amounts of water start there. Increase your water intake before moving further in the detoxification process.

As long as you are a smoker, you will need to pay special attention to your body's needs so it can continue to clean itself. Doctors of natural medicine use your general state of health, length of time, the quantity of smoking, and clinical symptoms to establish a safe and gentle ongoing detoxification program for you. If you have questions on how this might be done, please refer to Chapters 2-4 for further information—as they are referenced throughout this book and may help explain what a doctor of natural medicine might do for you.

Supplements

Typically, a good quality multiple vitamin and mineral formula provides what a human needs on a daily basis. Some people are better at getting these nutrients through diet while others need to supplement from a bottle. Most vitamins and minerals work better when complexed together, as they are in food.

With modern science, people can make whole food products and products which are complexed similar to how they occur in nature. Most doctors who specialize in natural medicine will use food as much as possible since the human body knows what to do with the substances food contains. But sometimes, especially when something like glutathione or N-acetylcysteine is needed, a supplement truly is the best way to get the proper levels.

Glutathione

Glutathione is the main antioxidant of the human body, and it is found in high levels in all cells. It is directly responsible for neutralizing free radicals from many different sources including chemical exposures. It is also responsible for regenerating vitamins C and E. When an antioxidant such as vitamins C or E binds with a free radical, the molecule stays bound to the vitamin until it is removed, in this case, by glutathione.

Glutathione is also an important cofactor for several antioxidant enzymes, meaning those enzymes wouldn't be able to function well, if at all, without it. It neutralizes free radicals that are made during phase I liver metabolism, transports mercury out of the brain and cells, regulates cell proliferation and apoptosis (meaning cell growth and cell death), and assists with mitochondrial function and mitochondrial DNA. This last action is very important because the mitochondria are the powerhouses located in every single cell except for red blood cells. Without adequate mitochondria function, you won't have enough energy to do everything you want to do in a day. For more information about glutathione, see Chapters 4, 6, 10, and 18.

Magnesium

Magnesium is critical to liver health and body detoxification. It helps move toxins through the digestive tract by supporting smooth muscles and promoting bowel regularity. Magnesium is needed to make glutathione and has been found to be especially protective of red blood cells, increasing their ability to deal with oxidative damage. Research has even found increasing your magnesium intake by 100 mg can reduce your chance of liver disease by up to 49%.

Magnesium also helps prevent damage caused by environmental factors such as toxins, heavy metals, and chemicals. In the form of malic acid, it binds to heavy metals, such as aluminum and lead, and carries them out of the body. For more information about magnesium, see Chapters 3, 4, 7, 15, and 18.

N-acetylcysteine (NAC)

NAC also deserves another mention in this section as it helps protect the liver from excess oxidative damage. Oxidative damage, over time or if there is just too much for the liver to process, overloads the liver and slows down the detoxification process. In addition to everything the liver does, it is also one of the primary producers of glutathione in the body. NAC is a precursor to glutathione, meaning it supports the body's production of its most important antioxidant. It also helps promote detoxification and helps protect cells by preventing cellular death through an increase of glutathione levels. For more information about NAC, see Chapters 4, 6, and 9.

B Vitamins

Part of detoxification is changing the toxins from one form to another, a process called methylation. Methylation—and therefore detoxification—are dependent on B vitamins to work properly. During detoxification, your liver and other detox organs convert and remove unwanted toxins from your body. For more information about B vitamins, see Chapters 4, 11-12, 14, and 17-18.

Vitamin C

Vitamin C recycles other substances such as glutathione and Vitamin E to keep the detoxification processes running. It also protects the liver from oxidation during both phase I and phase II detoxification in the liver, and assists in the direct removal of toxins. For more information about Vitamin C, see Chapters 3-4, 6-7, 9, 11, and 18-19.

Vitamin E

Vitamin E is a fat-soluble vitamin whose main role is as an antioxidant to pick up free radicals roaming around the body. It works in conjunction with Vitamin C and glutathione. Vitamin E is available in a supplement form. The best form is mixed tocopherols because this is how vitamin E is found in nature. There are food sources of vitamin E which include wheat germ, sunflower, safflower and soybean oils, sunflower seeds, almonds, peanuts/peanut butter, beet greens, collard greens, spinach, pumpkin, red bell pepper, asparagus, mango, and avocado. For more information about Vitamin E, see Chapters 4 and 11.

Botanicals

Burdock

Burdock (*Arctium lappa*) has been used for over 3,000 years as a medicinal herb. It has a rich history in traditional Chinese medicine where it is used as a blood cleanser. It has been used to help with skin conditions; it helps open up the pores to get things moving. Burdock is also nutritious and rich in minerals. Part of burdock's claim to fame is how it helps the body move toxins and protects the liver. It has been shown in animal studies to help protect the liver against damage caused by heavy metals like cadmium as well as alcohol and acetaminophen. Burdock has an anti-inflammatory action in the body which can help reduce pain from various causes. As an antioxidant, it helps scavenge free radicals. Burdock is also being studied for its anticancer qualities, its ability to help with blood sugar control in diabetes, and how it can support the immune system when dealing with viruses and other microbial invaders.

Burdock has caused rare cases of allergic reactions with topical oil use, so caution should be exercised by using a small amount at first or by talking it over with your holistic provider.

Milk Thistle

Milk thistle (*Silybum marianum*) is one of the oldest herbs recorded by humans for medicinal use. It is a powerful herb for supporting the liver because of its unique ability to protect liver cells from further damage. With liver damage, the cells of the liver suffer from reduced blood flow due to the inflammation in the hepatocytes (liver cells) crushing the blood vessels. Milk thistle helps prevent this type of damage. It even helps the liver regenerate itself and can help prevent fibrosis. This herb is an antioxidant. It slows down glutathione depletion, and it has been shown to improve liver enzymes over the course of a few months. Milk thistle is also anti-inflammatory. In general, milk thistle is considered to be a liver-protective herb.

Lifestyle

The basics mentioned in Chapters 3 and 4 are a great place to start if you need a reminder. The information in them is important to understanding the basics of creating health and is referred to often in this section. Included here are some extra and more in-depth things to consider while you are evaluating your lifestyle.

Diet

- Hydration with Water & Tea

  Water is important to overall health and well-being, and proper hydration is crucial to better health. It is also important in any conversation about forming any sort of detox routine—arguably, it could be the most important part. Whether you decide to buy a box of supplements off the shelf or participate in some sort of whole food cleanse, these all strongly recommend you incorporate lots of water into your day. Water is what adds liquid to your blood to carry vital nutrients and oxygen into your body, and it carries waste out. Those who have more adipose tissue can have a little less water in their bodies than that, but it is no less important. If you are someone who finds water tastes terrible, you can tailor it to your liking by adding some sliced lemon or lime to your glass. Other options include adding cucumber, blueberries, strawberries, or even using store-bought flavor packets.

  Tea is another great option to help you get enough fluids. Any tea works, but herbal teas without caffeine are more hydrating than those with caffeine. Caffeine is a diuretic which means that it will make you urinate more. There are many pre-packaged herbal teas available at your local grocery store, or you could visit a local tea/herb shop. A local shop will have people familiar with herbs at some level, and they may be able to help you blend a tea for your purposes. In addition to the herbs already listed in this chapter, you can consider including dandelion root, red clover, or nettle to your tea.

- Bieler's Broth

  Bieler's broth was developed by Dr. Henry G. Bieler. In many ways, Dr. Bieler was ahead of his time, believing diet either contributes to health or hurts it. This plant-based broth is very nutritive providing nutrients like B vitamins, and minerals like potassium, magnesium, manganese, and iron. Bieler's broth is also beneficial for internal organs including the liver and kidneys. It also works to restore the sodium-potassium balance in the body which can support adrenal function and other body systems.

  One of the purposes of the broth is to balance out the body's pH, as again, smoking increases the acidity of the body. This acidic environment is particularly damaging to the body's enzymes causing their shapes to change. This means your enzymes aren't working as efficiently or effectively as they should be. Being more acidic also means you aren't absorbing your minerals. This leads to mineral deficiencies over time. If you want to try Bieler's broth for yourself, you can find the recipe in the Apothecary section at the end of this book.

- Dietary Fiber

    Another way to support your body's detoxification is to make sure you are getting adequate amounts of fiber. Both soluble and insoluble fiber is important, but insoluble fiber is the main focus for detoxification support. One of the main pathways the liver uses to get rid of waste is through bile and stool. The liver uses bile and stool to get rid of certain wastes. Additionally, without proper fiber and hydration, constipation often develops. This should be avoided because if stool sits longer than it should in the body, the large intestine can reabsorb some of the toxins waiting to be excreted.

    Fiber has an impact on many areas of overall health; it is something everyone should focus on. It is possible to add fiber to your diet by eating more vegetables and whole grains. If that proves to be difficult, there are fiber powders on the market that can help. In general, you should strive for roughly 14 grams of fiber per 1000 calories eaten per day. How much is that, really? For example, 1 stalk of celery and 2 tablespoons of peanuts = 3 g of fiber. Additionally, avocados = 10 g fiber per 1 cup; beans = 8-9 g of fiber per ½ cup; chia seeds = 4 g of fiber per tablespoon For more information about fiber, see Chapters 3, 12-13, and 16.

Other Therapies to Consider

Castor Oil Pack

Castor oil packs were first discussed in Chapter 3, as a topical or external medicine. They can also be used to support your liver. The liver is responsible for breaking down hormones and excreting them through bile. Bile is a substance made in the liver and stored in the gallbladder. It is released into and used in the small intestine as a part of the digestive process of breaking down fats. This is also a way for the liver to get rid of substances your body doesn't need anymore, such as hormones. The heat of the pack will also stimulate blood flow. Complete instructions can be found in the Apothecary chapter.

Skin Brushing

Dry brushing the skin before showering or bathing is an excellent technique to get the lymph moving through your system. Moving lymph is important for proper detoxification. Detailed instructions are in the Apothecary chapter.

At-Home Contrast Hydrotherapy

This therapy is very tonifying and can increase the available energy to the entire body, especially the abdominal organs. This hydrotherapy will increase circulation to bring nutrients and oxygen in, and help to process waste products properly in their respective organs. The process can be done at home with a partner, or by yourself. It is important to combine this with a good diet and proper hydration, as this allows your body to detox and clean itself out. More information can be found in Chapter 4 and complete instructions can be found in the Apothecary chapter.

Sauna

Working up a sweat is important to detoxification because it gets things moving. Exercising is one way to do this, but another effective way is to use a sauna. Sauna has been used by humans for thousands of years in the form of sweat lodges, natural hot springs, etc. To put it simply, sauna involves sitting in a hot space to induce sweat for a set amount of time. This is done to encourage detoxification throughout the body. There are many different types of saunas from many different cultures. The main differences between types of sauna are the heat source and the type of humidity present.

Sauna has been shown to reduce free radicals, oxidative stress, and reduce inflammation. It also helps with blood sugar regulation by raising insulin sensitivity, supports heart health through increased nitric oxide availability, and exercises the vascular system. Research has demonstrated heavy metals such as lead, arsenic, cadmium, and mercury are eliminated through sweating. This makes sauna a powerful tool for smokers to help reduce their high toxin load.

Today, saunas are more commonly available than ever before. Most gyms and some hotels now offer sauna facilities. This trend is even reflected in medical offices and spa businesses that have sauna options for their clients to use. Another option is to purchase a sauna for your home. These can be semi-permanent structures that are small single-person units or room-sized permanently installed units. Saunas can have walls made of mud, salt blocks, or crystals like amethyst or rose quartz, or they can simply be made of wood. There are both wet and dry saunas. The most researched type of dry sauna is the Finnish sauna which has been around for over 2,000 years. This type of sauna harnesses dry heat and unlike steam rooms, also known as wet saunas, moisture and steam play no part in a Finnish sauna. The humidity is typically kept between 5-20% with a temperature between 80-100°C.

Caution: Before using a sauna, you should check with your health practitioner. You must also be well hydrated because, in a sauna, it doesn't take long to become dehydrated. Consider beginning with ten-minute sessions; you can incrementally increase your time to 30 minutes depending on your comfort and tolerance of the heat.

Fasting

Fasting is when you don't consume certain foods or food in general for a certain length of time. One study looked at men who fasted from sunrise to sunset, leaving them an eight-hour or less window to consume all their calories for the day. Researchers found participants had improved blood pressure with lower pressure changes. Almost two years after the study, participants retained better blood sugar control and reduced inflammation throughout the body. Intermittent fasting studies have demonstrated not only reduced free radicals and weight loss, but evidence that it lengthens your very existence by adding years to your life.

There are many different ways to fast depending on what your level of health is. Intermittent fasting is one option where food is avoided for 1-2 days a week, or for a certain span of hours during the course of a day. An example would be eating in a six-hour window during the day rather than eating at any time while awake. Alternate day fasting is where you eat one day and fast the second day. Another type of fasting is water fasting. It is also an option, but medical supervision is advised while water fasting, especially in smokers who already have a higher toxin burden.

An alternative way of fasting, especially for those who are more toxic or have a weaker vitality to start, is to stick to a plant-only diet for 3 to 5 days of the week. All processed foods, sugars, and meats are avoided during that time. This can be combined with intermittent fasting.

Before starting any fasting protocol, it is always recommended to speak with a qualified health professional. Sometimes, fasting protocols need to be altered to make sure the fasting experience is the best and safest possible. Fasting can release toxins which can cause symptoms including skin rash, gastrointestinal upset, mood swings, etc., and having your primary care physician or other healthcare professional on board is always the best idea. Always remember to drink adequate amounts of water while fasting, as water is crucial to flushing toxins out of the body.

Chapter 9:
Our Reproductive Parts

The cultural teachings from my Cherokee heritage share how the world should have balance, harmony, cooperation, and respect within the community and between people and all of nature. In this way, many lessons and traditions are passed from one generation to the next teaching us how to maintain natural balance, harmony, and health.

It's important to remember, especially for those considering having children, what happens now has an impact on the future generation. If parents take time to help prepare themselves physically and mentally for creating and nurturing a new life, it gives their offspring a healthier start. Both fathers and mothers contribute to this new life through their genetics which can be influenced positively by living a healthier lifestyle. In this way, we can be sure the human race itself has a better chance of survival in the future.

For those who won't be having any children or who are past this time in their life, keeping your reproductive system healthy impacts many other systems in your body. Sexual hormones influence cardiovascular health, bone strength, mental and emotional health, mood swings, cancer risk, etc. These hormones, including estrogen and testosterone, have their own ebb and flow throughout life, but this can be complicated by many factors.

The Reproductive System

The following section is a very brief overview of how the reproductive system works. There are many hormones at play in both men and women. These hormones are involved with reproductive health and other activities in the body, and information about these hormones will be mentioned where necessary.

Male

The male reproductive system is located more externally which includes the penis, scrotum, and testes. The penis is flaccid unless the male is sexually aroused. This triggers the penis to fill with blood and become erect, allowing penetration into the female reproductive tract for pleasure and/or reproduction. Below the penis is a loose sac of skin called the scrotum which houses the testes. The scrotum can raise and lower the testes to keep them at an optimal temperature for sperm production. The testes produce sperm and hormones including testosterone. On the back of the testes is an organ called the epididymis which matures, carries, and stores the sperm.

During sexual arousal, muscular contractions begin and send the sperm out of the epididymis into the vas deferens, a tube connecting sperm to the outside world through the urethra. Attached to the vas deferens are the seminal vesicles which nourish the sperm and assist with sperm motility. The urethra then passes through the prostate gland where fluid is added to the ejaculate which provides nutrients for the sperm. Ejaculation is when sperm and ejaculate exit the penis through the urethra.

In a healthy male, reproductive health means more than just achieving an erection during sexual arousal. Testosterone is involved with libido, bone health, muscle size and strength, bone mass, etc., and if this hormone is out of balance, these body systems are impacted. Fatigue, lowered strength, and weight gain are just a few symptoms that can result.

This section wouldn't be complete without the urinary tract organs as these two systems are so intertwined. In the male, there are two kidneys that filter contaminants, wastes, and nutrients from the blood to dispose of or recycle them. This creates filtered blood and urine. Urine then travels from the kidneys down the ureters to the bladder where urine is stored for excretion. When the bladder signals the nervous system it is full, urine will be released by the muscle relaxing and allowing urine to travel down the urethra and out of the body through the penis. This is the same structure that travels through the prostate where sperm and ejaculate fluids are added during sexual arousal.

Female

The female reproductive system is mainly located deeper inside the body. It consists of several different parts. The ovaries produce eggs which can be fertilized by sperm to create cells that, over roughly nine months, can grow into a tiny human. These small almond-shaped organs are also responsible for making sex hormones including estrogen and progesterone. Before possible fertilization, the egg leaves the ovaries and travels down the fallopian tubes toward the uterus. If fertilization has occurred, the egg will implant in the wall of the uterus and grow into an embryo; otherwise, hormone changes will trigger the menstrual cycle which involves the shedding of the uterine lining. Last but not least of the larger organs is the vagina which accommodates penial penetration. It is the gateway from the outside of the body to the uterus and maintains a more acidic environment to protect the body from microbes. The labia majora and minora protect the vagina's opening, and the clitoris, located at the anterior point where the labia minora comes together, is sensitive to stimulation and female arousal.

In a healthy female, the menstrual cycle is roughly 28 days in length though this can vary by being a few days shorter or longer. Days 1-14 are when estrogen is the more dominant hormone to signal the development of the egg, and days 15-28 are when progesterone is dominant, signaling the thickening of the walls of the uterus to support a fertilized egg's development. Menstruation should involve very little, if any, cramps, backaches/pain, food cravings, mood swings, etc. Sexual intercourse should also have little to no discomfort or pain involved.

The female urinary system is also composed of two kidneys, two ureters, and a bladder. Women don't have a prostate gland, so the urine exits the bladder through the urethra. The urethra is much shorter in women than in men due to anatomical distances.

How Smoking Damages the Reproductive System

In both men and women, cardiovascular health has an important impact on reproductive health. This is in part because of the circulatory effects of smoking but also because of the HPA axis in both men and women. The HPA axis refers to the communication between the hypothalamus, pituitary gland, and adrenal gland. The hypothalamus makes corticotropin-releasing hormone (CRH) which tells the pituitary gland to secrete adrenocorticotropin hormone (ACTH). ACTH signals the adrenal gland to make several hormones including cortisol and androgens, or sex hormones, like DHEAS, DHEA, androstenedione, and a small level of testosterone. If this communication pathway is interrupted, hormone balance and levels will be interrupted as DHEA is one of the primary precursors to estrogen and testosterone. Remember, a lot of damage accumulates as your overall toxic load increases over time.

Another way smoking negatively impacts men and women is through the effects it has on the urinary tract system. Smoking increases the risk of bladder cancer, incontinence (due to increased coughing due to smoking), and worsens interstitial cystitis, a chronic painful bladder condition. In men, studies have looked at the risk of developing benign prostatic hyperplasia (BPH) and smoking. BPH means the prostate gland is enlarged and hasn't been found to be cancerous. So far research has found little change in risk from non- and former smokers. Active smokers may have an increased risk, but this drops off when they quit smoking.

Male

In men, there is a dose-dependent effect on reproductive capacity. This means the more you smoke, the less likely your chances are of having a child. Sperm's mobility is lowered by nicotine and one of its metabolites, cotinine. They have also been linked to DNA damage in the sperm. Cadmium and lead, two heavy metals present in cigarette smoke, were also found to reduce sperm motility and the overall quality of the sperm.

Smoking also impacts hormone balance, though the degree of impact is still being debated and researched all over the world. Human studies have demonstrated mixed results, but one study by Svartberg, et al. included over 900 male smokers and noted total testosterone increased by 15% and free testosterone increased by 13%. Sex hormone binding globulin (this is what carries testosterone in the blood) was also increased. The authors of the study reported these hormone changes may not result in any sexual or clinical changes, though more research is needed for a definitive answer while animal studies over the years have definitely found significant hormone changes with testosterone and luteinizing hormone (LH). LH is the hormone that signals testosterone production. One hypothesis stemming from this research is that smoking may interfere with the hypothalamic signals to the pituitary gland or Leydig cells which produce hormones when signaled by the brain; however, research is still ongoing.

The last point which should be addressed for men is the increased risk of developing erectile dysfunction. The chances of developing this goes up in men who smoke 10 or more cigarettes a day, and the risk goes up the more years a man has been smoking. Stopping smoking can reverse some of this damage. For example, one study found heavy smokers who quit had a 50% improvement in erectile dysfunction six months later.

Erectile dysfunction also includes having an erection in the morning. A morning erection is a normal physiologic response during sleep as the parasympathetic system is more active. Morning erections can reduce in occurrence to the point where they no longer happen, and when this occurs, it should be taken for what it is, a serious warning sign of cardiovascular problems.

Female

In women, smoking can cause infertility at higher rates than in the general population. Overall, levels of estrogen and progesterone are decreased in smokers, impacting the entire reproductive system. Smokers have increased rates of spontaneous abortion, ectopic pregnancy, and it affects how the egg moves through the fallopian tube. Research shows oocytes, or eggs, move slower through the reproductive tract in smokers by impacting the movement of cilia and smooth muscle contractions in the fallopian tube. For women suffering from infertility who elect to use assisted fertility techniques, smokers were found to have a 50% reduction in embryo implantation and maintaining a pregnancy when compared to non-smokers. During egg retrieval procedures, fewer eggs and fertilized embryos were recovered as well. Studies have shown the overall egg (oocyte) reserve may be affected by free radicals from smoking. They cause damage to the DNA of oocytes, and this may affect the fertility of unborn female fetuses. More research needs to be done as there are some conflicting studies, but the potential impact on the human population could last for decades.

There is a strong causal relationship between problems in newborns and smoking mothers. Babies born to smoking mothers generally have a lower birth weight, and a much higher risk of birth defects including cleft lip, club foot, heart defects, and respiratory problems. There is also a lot of research demonstrating how it negatively affects behavior in these children. Some researchers have been actively studying long-term effects including a higher risk of developing obesity, diabetes, high blood pressure, and high cholesterol because of the lack of adequate nutrients and oxygen in utero. Smoking also affects DNA methylation which is responsible for regulating gene expression; these negative changes have been found to last into adulthood in children exposed to smoke before they were born.

How to Support and Heal the System

With reproductive system health, a good diet rich in vegetables, drinking water, and a basic exercise routine will go far to help you achieve your health goals. If you need to revisit Chapters 2-4 to remind yourself of the systems being discussed here please do so. With most of the therapies listed below, the key is to reduce the oxidative stress damage from the free radicals produced by smoking.

Supplements

With supplements, it's important to include a basic multivitamin that contains vitamins and minerals designed to help support overall health. Minerals are also essential to reproductive health; for example, magnesium specifically helps ensure good blood flow to unborn children, and it is also important to progesterone levels. Essential fatty acids (EFAs) are also important here as they are integral to the quality of the oocyte and sperm. These include omega-3s which have been shown to increase fertility in humans and other mammals.

CoQ10

Regarding reproductive health, CoQ10 has been found to be useful in both men and women. For men, CoQ10 is again protective against free radical damage which is one of the primary causes of damage to sperm. In mice who were exposed to cigarette smoke, CoQ10 was found to be protective of testosterone levels. CoQ10 also reduces DNA damage and apoptosis, or cellular death, in sperm.

The majority of research involving CoQ10 looks at women who are having fertility problems, especially in women who have a low ovarian reserve —women with fewer eggs. Low ovarian reserve could be due to age, toxin exposure, free radical damage, etc. Mitochondria, the energy-producing cells, are plentiful in oocytes, and by increasing CoQ10, this preserves what eggs women have left, and supports successful cell division in early embryos when fertilization occurs. For more information about CoQ10, see Chapters 4 and 10.

Vitamin C

Vitamin C deserves mention here because of its antioxidant abilities. Oxidative stress is one of the main causes of fertility issues due to smoking in men and women. In men, research has demonstrated a significantly lower amount of ascorbic acid in the seminal fluid of smokers. For more information about Vitamin C, see Chapters 3-4, 6-8, 11, and 18-19.

N-acetylcysteine

Again, it is important to emphasize antioxidant supplementation with smoking and fertility concerns. The reproductive systems of humans are vulnerable to oxidation, and as smoking creates reactive oxygen species supporting the body's innate ability to deal with oxidants is important. NAC is a precursor to glutathione production, the body's primary way of dealing with oxidation. This nutrient has been found to increase fertility in women, especially those with polycystic ovary syndrome and recurrent pregnancy loss. For more details on NAC, please reference Chapters 4, 6, and 8.

Botanicals

In this section, the information has been divided between men's and women's health so you can find what's most relevant to you and your health goals.

Men

Nettle

Urtica dioica, also known as stinging nettle, is a potent antioxidant, anti-inflammatory, and nutritive herb loaded with minerals such as calcium and iron. One study compared wheat, barley, and nettle root flour together for nutritional value, and nettle was found to far exceed the traditional grains. It has been used for allergies, urinary concerns including BPH, arthritis, and rheumatism among others.

Its antioxidant qualities are believed to positively impact male fertility. More research needs to be done, but one animal study found improved sperm quality and count in nicotine-exposed mice. The study also noted an increase in the diameter of the seminiferous tubules; this is where the sperm are produced and this may be a large reason why it is helpful in fertility cases. Nettle also appears to increase available testosterone by binding with sex hormone-binding globulin. Globulin is the protein that transports fat-soluble hormones through your blood. Nettle was also found to lower the conversion of testosterone to estrogen although it does this in small amounts. For more information about nettle, see Chapter 6.

Saw Palmetto

Saw palmetto (*Serenoa repens*) is a small palm tree that grows in several southeastern states in the United States. Its main habitat is in Florida because of the state's dry, sandy soils. Research has been ongoing for this herb specifically for BPH.

It is an anti-inflammatory herb that helps with prostate inflammation. Smoking has been shown to increase the risk of developing BPH, and part of this has to do with the inflammation caused by toxin exposure. After six months of regular saw palmetto usage in men with prostate disease, urinary symptoms showed improvement. Saw palmetto also has specific effects in the male reproductive system including inhibiting testosterone to its most active form dihydrotestosterone (DHT) in the periurethral region of the prostate gland. Inflammation in this region is primarily what affects urination. Saw palmetto doesn't decrease hormone levels in the blood including DHT, PSA (prostate-specific antigen which is what your doctor tests to check your prostate health), or overall testosterone levels.

The effective dose which is most supported by research is 320 mg daily. This herb is very safe but it tends to be slower acting than pharmaceutical options. If you have an enlarged prostate, saw palmetto may or may not decrease the prostate size; research opinions are at odds.

Additionally, taking nettle root and saw palmetto together helps improve prostate health even more, easing urinary issues such as blockages and slow urine flow. During one study, men between the ages of 50 and 88 took a daily dose of capsules equaling 320 mg of saw palmetto extract and 120 mg of nettle extract. This group was compared to finasteride, a medication commonly used for BPH. At the end of the two-month study, both the herbal and finasteride group had similar improvements in symptoms, though fewer side effects were noted in the herbal group.

If you find you are having any problems with urination, be sure to meet with your primary care physician right away as this may indicate more serious health concerns.

American Ginseng (root)

American ginseng (*Panax quinquefolius*) is one of the members of the ginseng family. It is common in traditional Chinese medicine. Ginseng translates into English as "main essence", and it is considered by ginseng botanical specialist Dr. Shiu Ying Hu to represent "the vital spirit of the earth dwell[ing] in a root. It is the manifestation of the spiritual phase of nature in the material form," as found in Donald Yance's book, *Adaptogens in Medical Herbalism*. Ginseng has been used for over 5,000 years in Asia for many different health concerns. American ginseng has traditionally been used for general weakness, irritability, as a mild nerve tonic, and to support digestion.

Research suggests ginseng is helpful with erectile dysfunction due to its antioxidant abilities and how it increases nitric oxide in the cardiovascular system. One study, which included forty-five men with moderate to severe erectile dysfunction, showed improvements in sexual performance and satisfaction after taking approximately 2.7 grams of Korean ginseng daily. Ginseng also helps regulate high cholesterol, an occasional contributor to erectile dysfunction. Ginseng has been shown to also increase libido in men and women, and improve fertility by increasing sperm production and quality.

Tribulus

Tribulus terrestris has been found to assist reproduction by improving the health of sperm. One in vitro study found tribulus extract increased sperm travel speed, motility, and viability. When used orally in a population of infertile men, tribulus increased dihydrotestosterone (the most active form of testosterone), lowered fat, and may have increased lean muscle mass. Sperm motility, concentration, and liquification (how fast ejaculate becomes a liquid) all significantly increased with tribulus as well although more research is needed. This herb also increases libido, potentially due to the effect it has on testosterone levels.

Tribulus contains zinc and calcium, and has antioxidant actions which may be partly responsible for its benefits to male fertility. Its main phytochemical protodioscin works on sertoli cells which helps mature sperm, increases immature sperm production, and growth of the seminiferous tubules where sperm mature. Research shows an effective dose of tribulus is between 500 mg - 1,000 mg daily.

Women

Black Cohosh

Black cohosh (*Actaea racemosa* or *Cimicifuga racemosa*) root, commonly called cimicifuga, has been used to support women's reproductive health throughout their life stages. Black cohosh grows in Canada and the eastern United States and was introduced to English colonists by Native Americans hundreds of years ago. Traditionally, it was used for infections, fatigue, kidney problems, labor, irregular periods, and premenstrual syndrome (PMS); in modern times, black cohosh has primarily been studied in relation to menopause.

Menopause has been found to occur earlier in smoking women, and the risk of having early onset menopause (before age forty-eight) is also higher. Black cohosh seems to raise low and lower high levels of estrogen, dilate peripheral blood vessels, and ease pain in the nervous system. These effects are believed to contribute to its effectiveness in supporting women through menopause. It can help with hot flashes, depressed mood due to menopause, low libido, or night sweats.

Many female smokers report increased hot flashes and more intense PMS, fibroids, and a number of other symptoms within the reproductive system. Research is ongoing and more studies need to be done, but using black cohosh at the proper dose seems to help lessen hot flashes, PMS, and other symptoms. Like with all medicine, it works very well for some and less well for others.

In general, research studies have demonstrated it can be safe to take this for up to twelve months consecutively at 160 mg daily. It can be taken once a day in a single capsule or two droppers full of a tincture form although the tincture is very bitter. In some women, this herb can cause side effects such as cramping, vaginal spotting/bleeding, a heavy abdominal sensation, headache, or even an upset stomach. If you have or have had breast cancer or liver disease, it's important to talk to a qualified health practitioner such as an herbalist or naturopathic doctor before taking this herb.

Avoid this herb during the first trimester of pregnancy.

Red Clover

Red clover (*Trifolium pratense*) is a common plant that grows in temperate regions all over the world except Southeast Asia and Australia. It has been used as a blood-building herb, to lower kidney inflammation, and for vaginal infections. Most commonly it is used as a respiratory antispasmodic for whooping cough, measles, etc., or as an anticancer herb. Additionally, it is anti-inflammatory and antioxidant which are important in helping deal with the negative effects of smoking.

Red clover is rich in estrogenic isoflavones (plant substances that act like estrogen to some degree in the body) which researchers believe is part of red clover's effective actions. It can be used during menopause; it has a modest effect on moderate to severe vasomotor symptoms like night sweats and hot flashes (especially when taken together with black cohosh). Red clover may help support memory, and it can also help with mental support by lowering anxiety during menopause. It appears to help strengthen bone health in post-menopausal women as well as has some metabolic effects; meaning, it may be helpful to women who have high cholesterol or insulin resistance (metabolic syndrome).

Chaste Tree

Vitex agnus-castus, commonly known as chaste berry or chaste tree, has been used for women's health by herbalists and natural health practitioners for decades. The dried berry from the Chaste tree is steeped in history, having been in use since ancient Grecian times, and it may have been in use earlier. It helps modulate reproductive hormones and has estrogenic properties.

Chaste berry has been used now and in the past to help with PMS symptoms. Research supports that the risk of developing PMS symptoms is higher in smokers than in non-smokers, and the severity of PMS appears to be dose-dependent; the more you smoke, the more likely you will have these symptoms. Since smoking also negatively influences the HPA (hypothalamus-pituitary-adrenal) system, this potentially makes this herb even more useful.

The effect of chaste berry is dose-dependent—the more you use the more it can inhibit prolactin, a hormone known for allowing mammals to feed their young milk. In fact, monks in the Middle Ages were said to use large amounts to inhibit sexual urges. Be sure to have a discussion with your doctor about this one if you have a history of ovarian, uterine, or breast cancer. Prolactin, a hormone affected by chaste berry, has over 300 physiological roles in the human body, because of this it is recommended to only take this herb for a few months at a time, then take a break. Since the dose of chaste tree varies tremendously depending on what it is being used for, it's best to consult with an herbalist or holistic practitioner before adding it to your health regime.

Red Raspberry

Red raspberry (*Rubus idaeus*) leaf has been used to support women's health at least as early as the sixth century. It is a potent uterine tonic that has been used to support pregnancy and childbirth; additionally, it has been used to help with severe dysmenorrhea (menstrual cramps). It is also a very nutritive herb and contains vitamins C, E, and minerals including calcium, magnesium, and zinc. It is also a potent antioxidant.

Animal studies show this herb has the potential to be incredibly useful. More testing still needs to be done in humans, but researchers found it improves memory, supports the thymus, liver, and uterine organs, as well as modulates hormones in perimenopause, potentially protecting the uterus from future negative tissue changes.

Red raspberry can be taken in a capsule or tincture form, but if you are able to take time out of your day to make tea, this one is great tasting. To make this tea boil water and pour it into a mug with 1-2 teaspoons of raspberry leaf. If tea isn't something you enjoy, you can still take it per manufacturer's instructions in capsule or tincture form.

Men and Women

Buchu

Buchu is an aromatic plant that grows mainly in South Africa and is said to be a magical herb. Buchu was a general name to describe any plant that could be dried and powdered, but today it specifically refers to either *Agathosma betulina* or *Agathosma crenulata*. Buchu is used for many different purposes including to help with rheumatic diseases, as a digestive tonic, and even to help lower fevers. Mainly, it is used for urinary tract health due to its diuretic (increases urination), antimicrobial, and anti-inflammatory qualities.

For men and women, it can help with urinary tract infections (UTIs) and it has been found to work against *Staphylococcus aureus* and *Klebsiella pneumonia*, two bacteria that can cause UTIs. Being anti-inflammatory, buchu helps increase urine flow. This helps flush the bacteria out of the bladder and urethra faster, thus reducing the length of infection. It has also been found to be helpful with kidney stones and hematuria (blood in the urine). It is a strong antioxidant—this is helpful to protect reproductive cells which is especially helpful in smokers.

This herb can be taken as a tea or tincture though tea-form appears to potentially be more anti-microbial than tincture form.

Hawthorn

Due to the high levels of proanthocyanidins and flavonoids in hawthorn, animal studies have demonstrated this herb has the potential to increase sperm quality and help modulate hormone levels in males. In females, it is protective of ovarian function and maintaining proper estrogen levels. As it is also protective of small vessels, it can be very useful in counteracting oxidation damage in the small vessels of the reproductive systems of men and women. For additional information about Hawthorn refer to Chapter 7.

Maca

A member of the brassica family, maca (*Lepidium meyenii*) has been used traditionally in Peru for more than two millennia. It grows in some of the harshest and coldest environments. Traditionally this herb is prepared by boiling which seems to activate some of its medicinal qualities. Maca can be used as a health tonic due to its nutritional benefits.

In women, it has been shown to help with post-menopausal depression and appears to help protect against osteoporosis. In men, it has been shown to have a small but very positive effect with mild cases of erectile dysfunction. It has also been shown to improve semen quality in healthy and infertile males by improving parameters like sperm count, motility, and in creating healthier sperm with fewer defects.

Overall, more research needs to be done in humans, but studies with the greatest effect show taking 3 grams daily for twelve or more weeks is most effective. There have been few safety studies, but traditional populations have consumed large amounts daily for years with little to no ill effects.

Lifestyle

Again, make sure you are taking care of your basic health foundations, as they are important for your reproductive health as well as your overall wellness. Drinking water and getting exercise moves your blood to bring nutrients and oxygen to where it needs to go. It also helps support the body with any detoxification processes going on (refer to Chapter 8 for more information). Sleep is also important as it allows your body time to rest, repair, and prepare for facing the next day.

Diet

The need for more high-quality vegetables and fruits in the diet cannot be emphasized enough. Antioxidants are highly protective for male and female reproductive cells, especially in smokers who are exposed to more oxidation damage. Fruits and vegetables also are high in fiber which helps bind toxins to carry them out of the body. Fish oil also deserves mention here because of the anti-inflammatory properties of omega-3.

For women, red clover and soy contain isoflavones which have estrogenic properties. In menopause when estrogen levels are lower, eating estrogenic foods like soy can sometimes help with symptoms like hot flashes or night sweats. It also seems to promote improved cardiovascular disease risk factors and improved blood sugar control.

In men, excessive intake of phytoestrogenic foods like soy may potentially lower sperm count. Roasted pumpkin seeds have been shown to be very supportive of fertility in men due to zinc, iron, and copper content; these minerals are necessary for optimal male fertility. The seeds have also shown promise in supporting prostate health in men with BPH.

While the diet is discussed in numerous chapters of this book, an in-depth discussion can be found in Chapters 3 and 4.

Other Therapies to Consider

Women

Seed Cycling

Seed cycling is a nutritional way of supporting the proper ebb and flow of hormones in a woman's monthly cycle. As mentioned at the beginning of this chapter, the average menstrual cycle is roughly 28 days with days 1-14 being estrogen-dominant, and days 15-28 being progesterone dominant. Eating different seeds during a woman's menstrual cycle encourages healthy levels of hormones at the appropriate times of the month.

On days 1-14 of a 28-day cycle, day one being the first day of your cycle all the way to ovulation, consume 1 tablespoon of either flaxseed or pumpkin seed. It is also recommended to take 1.5-2 grams of fish oil to support EPA/DHA fats which are important for overall health, including hormone balance. Research has found flaxseed can help regulate women's menstrual cycle as well. No women consuming flaxseed missed a period during this study, and hormone ratios between progesterone and estradiol (a type of estrogen) were found to be significantly higher as well.

On days 15-28, which is from ovulation until menstrual flow begins, eat 1 tablespoon of sunflower or sesame seeds. It is also recommended to take 500 mg of evening primrose oil which is loaded with GLA, another oil supportive of hormone balance. One study looked at sesame seeds in postmenopausal women and found daily consumption for 5 weeks significantly improved blood lipid ratios, increased vitamin E and overall antioxidant status, as well as SHBG, the carrier protein of sex hormones. Please note that women should adjust the length of seed consumption to match their particular cycle lengths such as a 26-day cycle or a 32-day length cycle.

Men and Women

Castor Oil Pack

Castor oil itself is very anti-inflammatory and pain-relieving when applied to areas of congestion like the liver. Adding heat helps drive this action deeper into the body. The heat will also stimulate blood flow to bring more nutrients and oxygen into the area as well as support waste removal through the kidneys and other organs. This process encourages healthy hormone balance.

To read more about the specifics of how to do a castor oil pack, please reference the Apothecary chapter. Also, you will find more information about castor oil packs in Chapters 3 and 8.

Constitutional Hydrotherapy

Constitutional hydrotherapy is useful to improve blood flow to the abdominal organs which includes the reproductive organs. As blood is the key to bringing nutrients in and toxins out, it makes sense why this would be included here. More information can be found in Chapter 4. You can find instructions on a home version of this therapy in the Apothecary section or find a practitioner that offers this in their office.

Abdominal Massage

Abdominal massage is another way to help support your liver by encouraging regular bowel movements. This helps avoid constipation which can alter hormone balance; if wastes don't pass out of the body in an adequate amount of time, the large intestine will reabsorb as much as it can. In this case, the hormones secreted by your liver will just be reabsorbed again.

Chapter 10:
Windows to the World

Humans live in a complex world that provides an immense amount of information to the senses. Whether someone has the use of all or just some of their senses, the body must take that information in, interpret it, and then respond accordingly. A great example of this is when someone touches a hot stove. The body feels heat (taking in information), and if it is too hot, a rapid series of events happens internally (interpretation of information), and without thinking about it, they pull their hand away (response). How quickly the hand is removed determines the severity of the burn.

The senses allow one to identify danger and pleasure and therefore assist in making decisions about how to respond. When the sensory system is functioning as it should, humans experience the world in a vibrant, rich manner. When damage has occurred to some part or parts of the system, the overall experience is less. A person may not see as clearly or hear all sounds. Perhaps their sense of smell is not as strong as it was or things have lost their taste. There are many ways to damage the sensory system, and smoking is one of them. Thankfully, there are also many ways to support healing in the body. In this chapter, the focus is on the five basic senses: sight, smell, taste, touch, and hearing.

The Sensory System

People are taught at a young age that there are five sensory organs (eyes, nose, ears, mouth/tongue, skin/nerves) and therefore five senses (sight, smell, hearing, taste, touch). In addition to the five senses you learned about in school, several more make up the sensory system:

- **Proprioception:** The awareness of where your body and its parts are
- **Vestibular sense:** The ability to sense your body movements in time and space
- **Internal senses:** Hunger, thirst, fatigue, internal pain, emotional disturbance, the need to empty the bladder or bowel, changing blood pressure, and changing pH levels
- **Extra-sensory perception:** Telepathy, precognition, intuition, distance viewing, etc.

As you can see, there are many more senses than just the basic five as most people are led to believe. And perhaps most intriguing is that all of the senses work together, share jobs, and can even take over for one another if needed. For example, you may already know how the taste buds and nose work together. We cannot taste well without the sense of smell.

Chapter 15 discusses the nervous system which carries information from the sensory system.

Seeing

The eye of an adult human is roughly an inch in diameter. Despite its small size, it is a critical organ to how humans perceive the world around them. The outer eye consists of the sclera which is the tough white part that gives the eye structure, the iris which is the colored portion surrounding the pupil or black center of the human eye, and the pupil itself. As light enters the eye, it passes through the cornea or outer lens of the eye, through the pupil, and then through the inner lens. Tiny muscles pull on the lens to focus the image being looked at on the retina in the very back of the eye. The retina is an extremely thin layer of cells made to sense light called rods and cones which allow humans to see in twilight and color respectively. The choroid is a structure directly behind the retina rich with tiny capillaries that provide oxygen-rich blood and nutrients to the retina. The optic nerve is directly connected to the retina, translating retinal information to the brain to interpret as vision. Inside the eye is a viscous jelly-like fluid that provides its shape. Other structures which are important to mention include the conjunctiva which is the very outer layer of cells covering the eye and the macula, a structure near the center of the retina which is responsible for the central vision that allows a person to read, write, focus on people's faces, etc., leaving the rest of the retina for peripheral vision.

Hearing

The ears are the part of hearing that is visible, but the inner workings of hearing are inside the skull. The outer ear has curves that help focus any sound waves into a more concentrated and easier-to-interpret signal. Sound waves travel down the inner ear canal where they encounter the tympanic membrane, otherwise known as the eardrum. This delicate membrane vibrates from the sound, causing movement in the tiny bones of the inner ear called the malleus, incus, and stapes. The stapes connect to the cochlea which is a curled snail-like structure filled with fluid. The vibrations then turn into waves in the fluid which triggers cilia or hair-like cells to create an electrical signal to the brain which is interpreted as sound. The semicircular canals are also in the inner ear, and these structures are responsible for detecting head position and maintaining balance.

Smell and Taste

This system includes the nose and tongue which are integrally related to each other. To start, let's focus on the nose. Humans are able to differentiate 10,000 different smells and, not surprisingly, the smell can change from person to person depending on how their brain interprets information. When breath enters the body, it begins its journey through the nares, or nostrils of the nose. Air swirls around three turbinates (superior, middle, inferior) which are scroll-like structures that increase surface area to provide rapid warming and moisturization of the air. This moisture protects the delicate olfactory tissue and cells in the upper nasal passage which detects molecules breathed in. Here the sinuses play an important role, helping keep the nasal passages moist as well as lightening the weight of the skull. The molecules are translated into electrical signals that travel to the brain and are interpreted as smell.

The mouth is the main passageway for food to enter the body. It contains teeth for chewing, but, most importantly, it includes the tongue. The tongue is a very muscular organ that helps direct food in the mouth so it can be thoroughly chewed. In the process of chewing, the food is covered by saliva which begins digestion and helps break food down into molecules. These molecules can be detected by the taste buds. There are three different types of tastebuds or taste papillae located on the tongue which can detect five main flavors sweet, bitter, salty, sour, and savory (umami); research is ongoing on a few different flavors including fatty, alkaline, metallic, and water-like receptors. A common misconception is that certain areas of the tongue detect certain flavors but this isn't true. The entire surface of the tongue can detect all flavors with bitter being more concentrated on the back of the tongue to protect from potential poisons which are perceived as bitter-tasting. It is estimated that humans can detect 100,000 different flavors when taste receptors and intensity are combined with smell, temperature, and food texture.

Touch

Finally, the skin is the largest organ of the body. This will be discussed further in the next chapter, so for now, let's focus on the touch receptors contained in the skin. These receptors can detect a wide variety of stimuli including variations of pain, pressure, vibration, and skin stretch detected by mechanoreceptors. Thermoreceptors detect variations in temperature, and nociceptors signal pain when it is damaging to the body. These receptors are located at varying depths in the skin, and they signal nerve impulses to the brain when they are triggered. These cells have varying sensitivity levels allowing a person to feel the breath of a baby on their face or a hard grasp of a hand on the arm or leg.

How Smoking Damages the Senses

Smoking has the potential to cause damage to the sensory system like many other systems of the human body. There is quite a bit of evidence and research about the damage caused to known sensory organs such as the eyes, nose, and mouth, but the other sensory systems should not be left out.

Eyesight

In general, smoking irritates all mucosal linings in the body, not just those in the lungs and blood vessels. Conjunctival mucosa is negatively affected by the chemicals and fumes present in cigarette smoke, making your eyes more red and watery. Additionally, smoking has been linked to causing ocular diseases for decades. Nicotine and other compounds which affect the cardiovascular system can cause spasming in the arteries of the eye, potentially leading to a lack of blood flow, retinal damage, and increased pressure in the structures of the eye as more damage to the blood vessels occur. Age-related macular degeneration, one of the leading causes of vision loss in modern societies, was found in one Danish study to increase the risk of developing this to be 2.5 times higher than in non-smokers. Cataracts are another main cause of visual impairment, and smoking increases the risk of not only developing cataracts but having a more severe case. Heavy metals like cadmium and lead have also been shown to accumulate in the lens of the eye not to mention the oxidation damage present, both of which negatively impact vision. It's also important to note color changes are possible in the eyes of 1/3 of all smokers.

Hearing

Hearing can also be damaged by smoking. Studies have shown the chance of having noise-induced hearing loss increases in smokers. Overall, the risk of hearing loss has been shown to be higher in current smokers than in those exposed to second-hand smoke or non-smokers. The risk increases with more cigarettes per day and with more packs per year smoked.

Taste

Smoking has been linked to a decrease in taste which is worse in those who smoke more heavily (10-20 or more cigarettes daily). The exact mechanism of diminished taste could be related to taste bud damage, a lack of minerals such as zinc, etc. Nicotine applications to the tongue have also been found to negatively impact taste. One study found once smokers quit, taste sensations began to recover after two weeks, but some former smokers had a reduction in taste for over one year. Smoking also greatly increases the risk of cavities and oral cancer, partly due to a higher chance of developing dry mouth. Physical changes such as a black, hairy tongue, or inflamed salivary glands can also develop as a result.

Smell

Smoking also reduces a smoker's sense of smell which has impacts on the overall quality of life, dietary choices due to food flavor, and it diminishes the ability to detect food that has gone bad. It also raises the risk of developing nasal and sinus pathologies, and with smell being integrally linked to memory, it may have effects on smell-linked emotions and memories.

Chapters 6 and 7 discuss how the cardiovascular system and respiratory systems are impacted by smoking. As blood flow and oxygen is reduced over time due to smoking exposure, this negatively impacts all organs in the body—especially the senses. Each sense is composed of highly specialized cells which require oxygen and nutrients to function optimally. This is displayed by reduced sensation in the skin, especially in the fingertips. As always, with any of the diseases mentioned in this book, the more cigarettes smoked, the higher your chemical and toxin exposure, and the more likely these symptoms will develop.

How to Support and Heal the Sensory System

Of course, the best way to restore health to any part of the sensory system is to quit smoking. But in the meantime, there is a lot you can do to support the health and function of the various organs and systems in your body.

Supplements

As always, it's important to make sure the foundational nutrients are covered. A multivitamin and multimineral are very useful, especially in smokers who may not have a diet high in vegetables. In general, making sure you have plenty of antioxidants such as vitamin C, vitamin E, zinc, etc., helps maintain your senses throughout your lifetime. Additional nutrients and supplements specific to the sensory system are listed below.

If you need a refresher on the basics of health before continuing, please refer back to Chapters 2-4.

Essential Fatty Acids (EFAs)

EFAs should be mentioned again due to their anti-inflammatory aspects. Regarding hearing, increased omega-3 consumption via fish and other foods has been linked to lowering the risk of hearing problems in older age. Research is both promising and actively ongoing for the effect of omega-3s on loss of smell and recovering smell from nasal surgery.

Regarding the eyes, one study looking at sets of twins with and without age-related macular degeneration(AMD) found that, although the risk of developing AMD increased in current and former smokers over non-smokers, adding in more omega-3s reduced their overall risk of being diagnosed with AMD. The amount of fat consumed in the diet was much less important when compared to the dietary omega-3 to omega-6 ratio, with the greatest risk reduction of developing AMD was found in those eating less omega-6s. To put this into a better perspective, the average American consumes somewhere between 1:15 and 1:50 omega-3s to omega-6s in their diet; this means most Americans have high levels of inflammation and are at a higher risk of eye disease because they eat too many foods rich in omega-6s. Additionally, research has also found omega-3s can help with dry eye syndrome including symptoms like burning and even inflammation in the eyelid. For more information on EFAs, see Chapters 4, 7, 9, 14-15, 17, and 19.

Lutein

Lutein is a special kind of carotenoid called a xanthophyll, meaning it has oxygen in its structure. This is part of what makes lutein such an important antioxidant in the eye. Lutein is concentrated in the macula of the eye as well as the brain, especially in infants and the elderly. It also has the ability to help filter blue light which ultimately reduces damage from sunlight and other harmful light sources. Other functions include activating the complement immune system, modulating inflammatory responses, and it is involved in the nitric oxide system which helps promote appropriate immune system responses.

Research is still ongoing, though lutein has been shown to help prevent AMD (mentioned above) which is a major cause of blindness in older adults. It can also help with cataracts as these develop due to oxidative damage to the eye lens. It is being assessed for its ability to help with retinitis pigmentosa, and retinopathy in premature infants, though again research is still being conducted.

It is known that lutein is absorbed in the gut with the assistance of enzymes that break down fats; any medications that interfere with cholesterol absorption or high-fiber diets can potentially lower the amount of lutein absorbed into your system. If you prefer a food route to add more lutein, look for vegetables like peppers, turnip greens, cooked spinach (16 mg in one cup), chard, and raw kale (11 mg in one cup); consuming these foods raw conserves more lutein although cooked foods typically still have some. Herbs like dandelion, basil, parsley, and paprika also have higher amounts. Research studies typically find benefit in adding at least 10-20 mg of lutein daily; check your supplements to see how much they have. Supplements are best absorbed when taken with meals while digestive enzymes are at their peak.

Glutathione

For smokers, smell and taste can be drastically changed. Part of this change is due to the role of glutathione and smell. Glutathione helps maintain higher quality enzymes in the nose which are required for accurate interpretation of smells. Research has found glutathione is needed for receptors to have the capacity to detect a wider variety of odors. This can also help with taste as the sense of smell and taste are so integrally linked. For more information on glutathione see Chapters 4, 6, 8, and 18.

CoQ10

Again, Coenzyme Q10, or CoQ10, is a lipid-soluble compound present in all human cells. Its main purpose is its role in the electron transport chain to make energy in the mitochondria, the organelles which create energy and heat that allows large mammals to survive and thrive. Its second main role includes its antioxidant abilities which are being actively investigated. It is protective of fats, lipids, and even the body's DNA; these functions are why it is so helpful in supporting and maintaining the mitochondria. Indeed, researchers have found when supplementing with CoQ10, energy levels and sensory function improves. For more information about CoQ10, see Chapters 4 and 9.

Botanicals

Anthocyanins

The main cause of most sensory damage is the high oxidation that occurs from cigarettes. If you choose to continue to smoke (or if you have recently quit), adding anthocyanins may help mitigate some of the damage. Anthocyanins are water-soluble pigments that give fruits and vegetables their vibrant colors, specifically pink, red, blue, and purple. Anthocyanins are part of a larger class of bioflavonoids that helps prevent oxidative damage in the body—bioflavonoids are explained in greater detail in the Botanical section of Chapter 7. These particular bioflavonoids are special because they can be absorbed whole through the intestinal tract; most polyphenols have to be broken down first. Anthocyanins are thought to make plants more adaptable to cold conditions, and they also improve the antimicrobial and antioxidant mechanisms in plants. For humans, anthocyanins are also very powerful antioxidants that work on all of the body's systems.

Anthocyanins are also great at protecting blood vessels from damage. Each human sensory system is dependent on capillaries and their ability to provide nutrients and oxygen as well as remove wastes and carbon dioxide. Because these vessels are so tiny, they can easily be damaged through unhealthy lifestyle choices. When capillaries are damaged, the circulation of all the nutrients that the body needs is negatively affected. A great way to protect the senses is to add in antioxidant-rich foods such as dark berries including blueberries, raspberries, blackberries, bilberries, black currants, etc.

Research on black currant has shown that supplements with 50 mg of the extract have increased blood flow in the extremities. Bilberry also has a lot of research showing it is protective to the eye, specifically the retina and lens. It can also help prevent cataracts which are caused by oxidative sun damage.

Additionally, red raspberry extract has been shown to protect the skin from UVB exposure, helping prevent DNA damage with its antioxidant and anti-inflammatory properties. Even a single serving can bring benefits. Whole foods are typically the best way to go, but if supplements are easier, you can use capsules or extracts of black currant, bilberry, or other whole-food berry-based supplements.

Green Oat

Green oat (*Avena sativa*) is a tall grass that has been cultivated for human consumption. Oats have been used by humans for thousands of years as a dietary staple which remained dominant until beer and bread became more popular. Traditionally, oats were used for sleeping difficulties, nervous exhaustion, and overall nerve weakness. It was also used externally to help support the skin with a wide variety of complaints including burns and eczema. Additionally, it has been used to support withdrawal symptoms from addictive substances including opium and tobacco.

Overall, this herb is great for many reasons, but it is included here because of its ability to help tonify the nervous system. Oats contain selenium which is an important cofactor for glutathione production to help deal with excessive oxidative damage caused by smoking. Oats also have more soluble fiber than other grains; this helps maintain a healthy gut microbiome, feeling full longer after meals, and slower stool transit to allow for more absorption of nutrients. Because of this, oats can help prevent cardiovascular disease and promote healthier cholesterol levels. It has also been shown to improve memory and concentration in stressful situations.

This herb can be drunk continuously throughout the day as a tea, used as a tincture, or it can be used topically in a bath or poultice for skin applications. It is very nourishing and supportive for your body as long as you are not allergic. For more information about green oat, see Chapters 14-15, and 18.

Ginkgo

Ginkgo (*Ginkgo biloba*) is an ancient plant species roughly 200 million years old, meaning it has survived since the time of the dinosaurs. It is often referred to as a "living fossil", and is the only living relative of its species. This was the first plant to germinate in Japan after the atomic bomb was dropped on Hiroshima in 1946. Medicinally, it has been used for over 2,000 years, and modern research supports its use for concerns like asthma, tuberculosis, stomach complaints, cardiovascular health, and to help support healthy blood sugar. Ginkgo biloba is a great antioxidant, and it works synergistically with other antioxidant herbs, adding to their mutual effectiveness. It's also antimicrobial, anti-inflammatory, helps balance cholesterol levels to healthier ranges, is liver and nerve protective, and may also be helpful with mood.

Ginkgo leaves and seeds can be used medicinally, but ginkgo extract, made from the leaves, has the most scientific support behind it. This herb is used for anti-aging, anti-tumor, and antioxidant purposes. It can also help increase blood flow through the small vessels in the body.

In modern times, it has been found to help with hearing conditions such as sudden hearing loss or damage due to ototoxic drugs. Ginkgo biloba was able to restore some sound perception by increasing hearing thresholds after a sudden decline in hearing. It may also help with tinnitus, especially ringing caused by cardiovascular disease, though research is mixed. If you decide to take ginkgo biloba, research shows taking 150-300 mg of extract daily is the most supportive.

Red Ginseng

Red ginseng, otherwise known as Korean ginseng (*Panax ginseng*), is an herb that has been prominent in Asian medicine for centuries due to its far-reaching health benefits. Korean history has documented its use for over a millennia. The word *panax* means "all cure", referring to its ability to have a positive effect on a wide variety of illnesses and diseases. The root of this plant is used medicinally once it is six years old. It is immune-modulating, an antioxidant, cancer-preventative, and it may even help improve blood glucose. With its antioxidant abilities, it has been shown to be protective of DNA, and to prevent LDL cholesterol from being oxidized, slowing down blood vessel damage.

It has also been studied as an addition to mouthwashes and rinses. One small study found a product with red ginseng extract to have far superior antibacterial qualities as compared to other leading commercial brands. Another study found it was helpful with dry mouth in post-menopausal women.

If this herb is one you'd like to try, research shows taking 300 mg - 600 mg of red ginseng can help support oral health. You can also use a mouth rinse with ginseng or use it in tincture form and add it to some water to make your own mouthwash. This herb has been shown to be safe in humans but for some may cause heartburn, trouble sleeping, or increased hot flashes.

Lifestyle

Diet

As always, it is best to maintain a well-balanced diet. Eat a variety of fruits and vegetables including all the colors of the rainbow, to get vitamins, minerals, and antioxidants. The fresher the better! These foods serve as a cornerstone of a healthy diet. Additionally, make sure to get enough protein. Proteins provide amino acids for the body to use when building and repairing muscles and bones, when making hormones and enzymes, and can be used as an energy source. Fiber is important to help eliminate toxins, and healthy fats are important for cells to talk to one another and for hormonal health, among other things. Remember you are built out of what you eat. The more real food you eat and the more unprocessed your diet, the healthier you can become. If you'd like more detailed information, review Chapters 3 and 4.

Exercise

- Olfactory Training

    This is the use of exercises to help improve your sense of smell. Some new research has found that in patients who had lost their sense of smell due to COVID-19, retraining using different odorants for up to three months or more was successful in helping the majority of people get their sense of smell back. Since many smokers also lose their sense of smell, this therapy appears promising.

    In order to do olfactory training, you need the basic four scents: rose, eucalyptus, lemon, and clove. You will need four brown glass jars or bottles. Put a cotton pad in the bottom of each jar, then drop pure essential oils (roughly 1 mL of oil) onto the cotton. This will hold the scent for quite some time.

    The next step is to do the training itself. It's necessary to do this daily by spending at least 20 seconds inhaling each scent and has to be done without a break during that 20 seconds. The entire procedure should be done twice a day for the greatest effect. Depending on the cause of the lack of smell, approximately 6 months - 12 months of training shows the best improvement.

- Eye Exercises

Vision therapy has been shown to be effective for diagnoses including reading problems, focusing, convergence, and divergence. When the eyes aren't working together the way they should, this therapy may offer benefit. In today's highly technological society, people are commonly focusing on a screen close to their face whether it's a phone or otherwise. Without regular eye breaks, the muscles in your eyes won't work effectively over time. In smokers, the eyes are under additional strain due to high toxin exposure and oxidation, both of which contribute to eye issues.

These exercises are not replacements for regular eye checkups with your doctor, but they can help strengthen and maintain eye health. Be sure not to do too many repetitions at a time initially as you are working out a muscle just like any other. Doing these 3-5 times per week, with no more than once daily is recommended. Overdoing it could cause eye strain and pain.

1) Focus in General

   One way to exercise your eyes is by focusing. Take your index finger and hold it close to your face and focus on it. Slowly move your finger away from your face while maintaining focus on your finger. Once your arm is extended, focus somewhere in the distance beyond your finger, then focus on your finger and maintain that focus as you bring your finger back toward your face. Do this for 30-60 seconds.

2) Distance Focusing

   For this exercise, begin by holding a pen or other object in your hand. Focus on the object for several seconds, then change focus and look at something 10-20 feet away for several seconds. Continue focusing near and far for five repetitions.

3) Figure 8

   This exercise involves staring at a wall or the floor roughly ten feet away from you. Draw an imaginary figure eight with your eyes in one direction for 30 seconds. Take a brief pause, then do figure eights again for another 30 seconds, moving your eyes in the opposite direction. These can be done several times a day for the greatest benefit.

- Isometric Exercises

   An isometric exercise is one in which you contract your muscle but do not engage the joints or lengthen the muscle. This type of exercise has many benefits including activating muscle fibers and increasing electrical flow, in turn, this can help with overall nervous system communication. There are many self-help learning opportunities online, in books in the library, and with personal trainers. More information about exercise can be found in Chapter 3.

Other Therapies to Consider

At Home Hydrotherapy

Enough can never be said about water therapies and how supportive they are of your overall health and well-being. This is very tonifying to the entire body including the microvasculature which brings blood to all of the sense organs. Again, this will increase circulation to bring nutrients and oxygen in, and help to process waste products properly in their respective organs. Remember it's important to combine this with a good diet and drinking plenty of water with this allows your body to detox and clean itself out over time. This therapy can be done at home with a partner, or you can do it by yourself. More information can be found in Chapter 4 and complete instructions can be found in the Apothecary chapter.

Skin Brushing

Skin brushing is included here as it is a great way to stimulate and remove dead cells from the skin and move the lymph. Dry skin brushing is best done before a shower or bath. You can find more detailed instructions in the Apothecary section.

Chapter 11:
Beauty is Not Just Skin Deep

It's possible to tell, just by looking at someone, how healthy they are or are not. Looking healthy and fit is so important to humans that people around the planet spend billions of dollars every day on products, therapies, and lifestyles to keep themselves looking their best. They smear creams and oils on their skin, color and condition their hair, paint and sculpt their nails, and shave, bleach, and pluck unwanted hair from places. Humans are obsessed with how they look to others. This obsession is driven by the biological instinct to reproduce and continue the species.

It is not just looks that matter. The color and quality of the skin, the condition of the hair, the health of the nails, and the shine of the eyes are all indicators of vitality, something that attracts the opposite sex. This increases the potential to reproduce. Healthy and intact skin helps to protect the internal parts of the body from water loss, invasion of unwanted organisms, and starts making Vitamin D from sunshine. Head and body hair play a role in the sensory experience and nails protect the tips of your fingers and toes.

This chapter focuses on how smoking damages the skin, hair, nails, and glands, all parts of the integumentary system and what can be done to support that damage. If you need help remembering the part played by the nerves in the skin, please refer back to Chapter 10.

The Integumentary System

The primary purpose of the integumentary system is to protect the body from things such as ultraviolet light, dirt/dust, microbes, etc. This system includes the skin, hair, nails, the layer of tissue under the skin referred to as the subcutaneous layer, and the glands held within the skin. The subcutaneous layer is what keeps the skin attached to the muscles and organs inside the body. Each part contributes to survival, for example: hair keeps heat in and protects delicate structures such as the eyes, the subcutaneous layer has fatty tissue which also helps hold in heat, and nails which allow greater dexterity with picking up small objects and protect fingers and toe tips from injury.

 The skin, which is considered the largest organ in the human body, helps regulate body temperature by insulating and cooling via sweat, sensing the outside world, and by synthesizing Vitamin D and some B vitamins. There

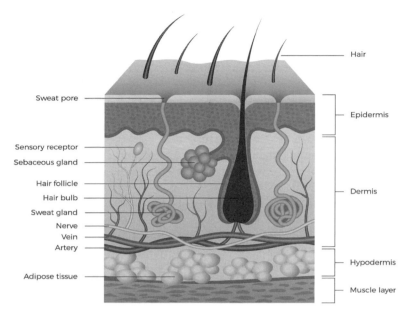

are two layers to the skin called the epidermis or outer layer of skin and the dermis (aka the subcutaneous layer). The epidermis also has layers, but more importantly, it is made of specialized waterproof cells called keratinocytes. The epidermis doesn't have its own blood flow. Because of this, it is dependent on the dermis for providing nutrients and oxygen. The dermis is the most active layer of the skin, and it contains blood vessels, nerves, hair follicles, smooth muscle, and lymphatic vessels.

Also embedded in the dermis are the glands. Several types of glands enhance the dermis' ability to protect us. Sudoriferous glands are sweat glands that help cool the body down if it gets too warm. Sebaceous glands create an oily substance that helps moisturize the skin, creating a barrier to keep germs, water, and dust outside of the body. Ceruminous glands make cerumen, the waxy substance in the ears, which helps protect the hearing by keeping the canal free of debris and bacteria as well as keeping the eardrum moisturized. Mammary glands produce milk for feeding infants.

The skin is full of collagen and connective tissue. This provides strength, durability, and flexibility to the skin, allowing us to scrape against something and not always sustain an injury. Melanin is also present in the skin and gives the skin pigmentation or color. The nails and hair are mainly composed of keratin, a specialized form of fibrous protein which provides structure in various areas of the body.

How Smoking Damages the Integumentary System

Most people are able to recognize smokers or former smokers by their gravelly voices and the appearance of their skin. Smoking can cause a yellowish or grayish complexion and increase wrinkles at younger ages because tobacco interferes with collagen development and repair of the skin. In people who smoke forty or more packs a year for five or more years, the skin loses a significant amount of elasticity which may explain early and increased wrinkles and brittle nails. Tobacco can also stain the skin and nails though this discoloration tends to improve when you quit.

Some research has found that smoking affects the structure and thickness of the skin when comparing smokers to non-smokers. It also delays wound healing, partly due to its impact on circulation in capillaries, and partly due to decreased fibroblast activity (cells that help with tissue repair). Some surgeons refuse to do surgeries on smokers if they won't quit because of the increased risks of wound complications. Smoking also increases the complications and severity of psoriasis, raises the chances of having contact skin allergies, and is a well-known risk factor of hair loss.

Additionally, it significantly increases the risk of developing skin cancer including squamous cell carcinoma and basal cell carcinoma. Due to the exposure of the oral mucosal tissues to the smoke, there is also a higher risk of oral squamous cell carcinoma which has a survival rate of less than 50%.

How to Support and Heal the Integumentary System

It is true, part of caring for yourself can involve looking your best, but so much of the damage from smoking can be unseen for many years. This system, like all the systems, is capable of great healing once the damage stops. Until you are ready to take that step, do what you can to support a healthier state. If you need to, refer back to Chapters 2-4.

Supplements

Vitamin C

Vitamin C is a potent antioxidant present in many different body systems but it has an especially high concentration in the skin. This vitamin is important for the body to heal wounds properly, mainly due to its critical role in building and maintaining elastic fibers in the body. Collagen is built from three protein chains, and Vitamin C is what holds these chains together. Without adequate

Vitamin C, which is often deficient in smokers, it can cause dental problems, poor wound healing, and bruising among other symptoms. For more information about Vitamin C, see Chapters 3-4, 6-9, and 18-19.

Amino Acids

Concerning humans, there are twenty amino acids critical to health—nine of which are essential. Essential amino acids must be absorbed through diet and include histidine, isoleucine, leucine, lysine, methionine, phenylalanine, threonine, tryptophan, and valine. Amino acids are the building blocks of proteins which are important to many different critical health functions. Regarding the skin, a few amino acids have been found to be especially helpful.

Arginine helps regulate the skin repair process by increasing nitric oxide, shifting the repair process from inflammatory stages, and has been shown to increase collagen repair in acute skin wounds. Another amino acid, methionine, has been shown to improve skin barrier functions by tightening the junctions between cells.

Vitamin E

Vitamin E has been used to support skin health for over fifty years. It is a potent antioxidant that helps protect cell membrane integrity, has also been shown to protect the skin from UV radiation, and has antitumor qualities.

Vitamin E can be taken internally as a supplement, but it can also be applied directly to the skin. Please note it isn't advised to apply it to the skin before being exposed to direct sunlight for a long length of time as this may be potentially damaging. As a result, using Vitamin E as part of a nightly skin routine is highly advisable.

Using a mixed tocopherol supplement is best as this is how vitamin E occurs in nature. Most supplements contain only alpha-tocopherol which is often made in a laboratory setting. To supplement this in your diet, sunflower seeds, almonds, hazelnuts, and olive oil contain tocopherols. You can also add tomatoes, avocados, spinach, asparagus, Swiss chard, or broccoli. Vitamin E is safe topically and is considered well-tolerated if taken internally. Talk to your doctor before taking Vitamin E supplements internally if you are taking blood thinners as both together may affect clotting. For more information about Vitamin E, see Chapters 4, and 8.

Minerals

Making sure you have a multimineral in your supplement regimen will help preserve and potentially restore your skin health if it has been damaged by smoking. For example, zinc has been shown to have antimicrobial qualities, especially when applied to the skin in a sunblock form, and protects from sun damage. Selenium also protects the skin from UV damage, and copper has been found important to collagen synthesis in the skin. It's best to take a multimineral with food to help improve absorption. More information about minerals can be found in Chapters 3 and 4, and are also discussed throughout most chapters of this book.

Botanicals

Calendula

Calendula officinalis has been used since the Middle Ages in herbal medicine. It was also used during the American Civil War in antiseptic and anti-inflammatory balms and creams. Traditionally, it has been used for gastrointestinal complaints, menstrual pain, and many different skin complaints. In modern times, calendula has been used in animal studies by exposing rats to cigarette smoke for an hour twice a day; the animals then either received water or calendula extract once a day. Results from this study indicate calendula is a potent antioxidant and may be protective from cigarette smoke's damaging effects when taken internally.

Calendula can be used topically as well, which is where it really shines. It has been used in wound healing, especially in inflamed wounds, for hundreds of years. One small study noted a 90% rate of wound closure versus a roughly 50% wound closure eight days after receiving a wound. It was also found to speed the healing of lower leg ulcers and other wounds. Additionally, it is antimicrobial, and it will help kill off foreign microbiomes in a cut.

If you'd like to add this to your daily routine, you can enjoy a cup of warm or cold tea, add the petals to your salad or sandwich, use a tincture or capsule form, and/or use it topically. For more information about calendula, see Chapters 6 and 16.

Gotu Kola

Gotu Kola (*Centella asiatica*) in addition to being helpful for the respiratory system, has anti-inflammatory and pain-reducing properties. It's also able to protect against and potentially reduce mitochondrial damage. Remember mitochondria are the cellular powerhouses. As with most herbs, gotu kola also has antioxidant properties which help protect smokers from the damage of smoke inhalation. Research demonstrates gotu kola helps heal wounds by increasing collagen production. Additionally, it has been found to help reduce anxiety and depressed mood, help with COPD and other lung conditions, and improve liver fibrosis.

Gotu kola is generally well tolerated; however, it is recommended to have a conversation with your doctor before adding any new supplements. For more information about gotu kola, see Chapters 6 and 15.

Dark Berry Extracts

Dark berry extracts contain polyphenols which are very beneficial for overall health and were previously discussed in Chapter 7. They help protect DNA from damage, protect mitochondria, help reduce or prevent fine lines and wrinkles, and they are loaded with antioxidants. Again, it's important to realize a lot of damage from smoking is due to oxidative damage. Berries are high in antioxidants due to the presence of flavonoids like anthocyanins and phenolic acids. Examples of dark berries include blueberries, blackberries, mulberries, raspberries, etc. In addition to getting fresh berries when they are in season, frozen berries are a great option if they are flash-frozen at their peak freshness.

Lifestyle

Diet

It will always be important to remember you are what you eat. Antioxidants that come from fresh and colorful fruits and vegetables are center stage in regard to skin health. These molecules play a critical role in keeping your integumentary system healthy. These foods are also loaded with fiber which helps improve your body's ability to detoxify, maintain a healthy hormone balance, and have a regulated digestive tract with a healthy gut microbiome, among other things.

There are a few foods and food additives you should try to avoid. Fried foods are pro-inflammatory as the oils used are oxidative and tend to be omega-6 heavy oils. When cooking at home, use anti-inflammatory high heat tolerant cooking oils like safflower. Additionally, it's vitally important you decrease your intake of added sugar. Research has shown high glucose in the blood impairs keratinocytes, the skin's cells that repair and maintain healthy skin. Lowering your intake of food preservatives as much as possible to decrease the toxic load on your liver is also recommended.

Water is critical to your overall health, especially the skin. When your body is dehydrated, it shows in your skin: drier, itchier skin, more frequent appearance of fine lines, dull appearance, slower wound healing, etc. It's important to maintain proper hydration by following this general rule: drink 1.2 your body weight in ounces of water. For example, if you are 150 lbs you would drink 75 oz of water. This must be adjusted for each person depending on how active they are, medications, perspiration, kidney health, and diet. Make sure you are getting water with minerals in it. If you use reverse osmosis (RO) water then add minerals after filtering. Minerals in water help the body absorb water better, making sure it gets into the cells where it's needed.

While the diet is discussed in numerous chapters of this book, an in-depth discussion can be found in Chapters 3 and 4.

Exercise

Exercise is very supportive of every system in your body, and arguments can be made that this is one of the most health-supporting habits you can build into your lifestyle after diet and water intake. The key here is to just increase your movement little by little on a daily basis, especially if you aren't able to commit to an entire exercise routine. Health professionals recommend at least 30 minutes of movement 3 times a week, but parking farther from the store, going up and down the stairs a few extra times, or doing squats and push-ups for 5 minutes a day all increase your daily movement.

So why is exercise good for skin health? Remember, circulation is the key to health, and movement helps increase your circulation. Blood is what carries oxygen and nutrients into cells as well as carbon dioxide and toxins out. More information about exercise can be found in Chapter 3.

Other Therapies to Consider

As mentioned in previous chapters, constitutional hydrotherapy and skin brushing will help increase circulation. Skin brushing can also help with detoxification in the skin. Instructions for these therapies can be found in the Apothecary section.

Oil Cleansing

Oil cleansing has been used in many cultures for hundreds of years as a way to maintain skin health. In the United States, most commercially available skin care products tend to be drying because of the belief that oil on the skin causes acne and blemishes. You should also know that if the skin is too dry, it can't protect effectively from the damaging effects of UV radiation, germs, or be as resistant to physical damage. Oil cleansing has been found to help remove oil and non-oil-based make-ups, dirt, and sebum from the skin. There are many different oils that you can use, so be sure to choose one that would be most beneficial for your individual skin type. Additionally, adding liquid Vitamin E to your oil blend can add extra benefit.

Here are a few oils which you can consider adding to your daily regimen.

- Olive oil is a medium-weight oil, is anti-inflammatory, promotes skin healing, and may be beneficial for drier skin types
- Sunflower oil is higher in linoleic acid, and it hydrates the skin right away without inducing any redness
- Coconut oil is a thinner oil, and it is very nourishing and protects against UV radiation; it doesn't hydrate the skin as well as other oils, so this may be better for oily skin or as a component to your oil blend
- Safflower oil is anti-inflammatory and has analgesic properties; more research is needed to see how it holds up clinically with inflammatory skin conditions
- Additional oils to consider include grapeseed, argan, soybean, borage, avocado, jojoba, peanut, sesame, castor, etc.

Directions for Oil Cleansing:

1) Doing a patch test on your skin first to make sure you don't have an allergic or inflammatory reaction is best. Do this by applying oil to the area behind your ear or your jawline. Wait 24 hours after the application to see if there's any kind of reaction.

2) After testing, pour 1-2 teaspoons of oil into your hand, then proceed to massage the oil into your skin. Do this for several seconds to allow the oil to penetrate your skin to lift up any dirt or oil present. Do this BEFORE wetting your skin with water.

3) Next, remove the oil with a warm washcloth. Be gentle while doing this so you don't irritate your skin. If you wish to leave some of the oil present on your face, rinse with warm water instead and pat your skin dry.

4) Apply moisturizer if needed.

This can be done once a day, or a few times a week as a special addition to your skin care regimen. Sometimes oil cleansing can cause a purging reaction where you may have a slight breakout as the skin detoxes itself—this may occur during the first one to two weeks. If you notice any itchy, raw, or inflamed skin, this is a sign of a reaction, and you should discontinue oil cleansing until you talk to your doctor or dermatologist about it. Sometimes delayed negative reactions occur despite doing a patch test while your skin is adjusting to the oil.

Mud Therapy/Peloid Therapy (Mud Packs)

Clays and muds have been used by humans since before recorded history began. The first written history we have is from Mesopotamia in 2500 BC which mentions using clay for helping staunch bleeding wounds and to encourage wound healing. Mud packs were recorded as being used in European spa resorts in the 18th century up through current times. There are many, many different types of muds and clays that can be used externally to support the skin.

In modern times, mud packs have been found to be very anti-inflammatory as well as pain relieving, and they have specific beneficial applications in cases of osteoarthritis and rheumatoid arthritis. One study looked at patients who had a yearly mud pack; hormones were more balanced (lowered stress), inflammatory markers decreased, and antioxidant responses increased. Mud packs also have nutritive minerals, some of which can be absorbed through the skin. Another study reported an increase in microcirculation which is helpful as circulation brings oxygen and nutrients to the skin and carries toxins and carbon dioxide out.

Additionally, mud and clays are very absorptive, meaning they will absorb toxins and microbes to help eliminate these elements from the skin's surface. Some mud also helps maintain a more alkaline balance in the skin, helping protect it from bacteria and viruses. Both of these effects can ease symptoms caused by oily skin, acne, psoriasis, or eczema.

In the smoking population, the skin has to deal with more toxins and oxidants than non-smokers. Clay can be a great at-home tool to help moisturize and balance your skin's overall health and appearance. When you are doing it for yourself, do some research into what type of clay will support your skin health goals. Bentonite can be firming and moisturizing, French green clay has been shown to be antibacterial, etc. These packs can be applied warm or cold, and to any area of the skin except sensitive parts such as the genitals, eyes, ears, nostrils, and mouth. Check the Apothecary chapter for a DIY Mud Pack.

Note: Some edible clays exist, but are beyond the scope of this book. As mineral and heavy metal content vary greatly from clay to clay, the use of clay internally cannot be condoned unless you are under the care of an experienced holistic practitioner familiar with clay and its uses.

Bentonite Clay

Bentonite clay is named after Fort Benton, Wyoming, where this particular clay has the largest deposits discovered in the late 19th century. There are records of bentonite being used medicinally for potentially thousands of years. Michel Abehsera in his book *The Healing Clay* states Native Americans called bentonite clay *Ee-Wah-Kee*, meaning "The Mud That Heals". It is an antimicrobial clay that can be used internally or externally to support overall health and well-being. Internal use should be overseen by a trained professional.

Externally, it has been found to be very soothing to the skin with slow wound healing, skin inflammation or irritation, and it has also been found to help reduce toxins. To use this topically, you can make a paste with bentonite clay and water or jojoba oil to apply topically as a mask to your face or other areas of skin that are concerning you. It can also be used as a homemade or premade toothpaste which can help remineralize teeth, as well as help maintain a healthy bacterial population in your mouth.

Facial Exercise

For centuries, people around the world, especially in some Asian cultures, have used facial exercise, also known as face yoga, as a way to reduce their appearance of aging. It works by strengthening the muscles underneath the skin, to tighten the skin, and reduce the appearance of aging. There is some research out there supporting this, though most of the studies are small and are based on the subjective opinions of the patients themselves. One study in 2018 took before and after photos for comparison, and they found positive improvements in all subjects who completed the study with fuller upper and lower cheeks.

1) Facial Tapping

    This works to increase circulation in your skin. Start at your forehead and use your fingertips to rhythmically tap your skin, moving down to your jawline. Next, tap the front of your neck and across your shoulders, moving up the back of your neck to the base of your skull. Finally, rub your hands together to create heat, cup your hands over your face, and breathe deeply for several breaths.

2) Smoothing Your Brow

This is helpful as many people hold tension in the forehead. Place your fingertips of both hands in the center of your forehead. With a gentle pressure, pull your fingers outward towards your temples. Release your fingers, and repeat this for 30 seconds.

3) Eye Circles

This may help relieve puffiness around your eyes. Be sure to use a very light touch. Start by placing your index fingers at the inside of your eyebrows, then gently tap outwards towards your temples. Press gently into your temples for a few seconds, then continue tapping above your cheekbones to the inner corner of your eyes. Repeat for 30 seconds.

Additionally, you can work to add more conscious smiling to your day. In addition to lightening your mood and increasing a general feeling of well-being, it also strengthens facial muscles as noted above.

Sole

Making sure you have adequate minerals in your foods and water is important to maintaining proper skin hydration. One easy way to do this is by adding *sole*, salt water made from Himalayan salt. The water naturally concentrates the salt, making it roughly 90% salt and 10% trace minerals.

To do this, use a small glass jar, 8-12 oz, with a lid. Add food-grade Himalayan salt chunks to the jar, squeezing as many in as will comfortably fit. Add filtered water to the jar so it just covers the salt, and let it sit for 24 hours.

To use it, take ¼ teaspoon of the sole and add it to an 8 oz glass of water. It will taste slightly salty for the first few days. It's best taken in the morning as it will encourage regular bowel movements as well as help regulate your thirst throughout the day. If you tend to be very thirsty throughout the day no matter how much water you drink, or if you tend to never drink water, this can help encourage a proper thirst stimulus.

Chapter 12: Wipeout!

The anatomy and physiology of humans is ideal for a creature on the go! Humans run, walk, lift, push, pull, sit, stand, dance, twist, bend, think, and so much more every day. This ability to constantly move and be full of energy is made possible by processes that run behind the scenes, meaning, we do not feel nor are we aware of all the things happening in the body that result in this energized feeling. However, most humans can feel the slightest drop in energy very quickly. When the body is healthy enough, these energy drops are fleeting; though, the more demand we put on our body, the more time it needs to recover. Again, when the body is healthy enough, it self-heals, recovers, and returns to a normal state of having more than enough energy to get us through the entire day.

As discussed, there are many pieces, parts, and processes that lead to a healthy enough state. Feeling energized is no different. The body needs proper circulation, strong lungs, communicating nerves, good GI function, healthy adrenals and thyroid, sufficient nutrition and hydration status, quality rest, physical conditioning, toxin elimination, a clean environment, and mental and emotional balance. When all of the above are in working order, a person is living a life without the symptoms of illness.

This chapter focuses on the adrenal and thyroid glands. Smoking can affect the function of these glands and supporting these systems can set you on the path to better health.

The Adrenal and Thyroid Glands

One of the reasons why the adrenals and thyroid are discussed together in this book is that they work in tandem with one another for many things in the body such as metabolism, immune function, blood pressure, and the stress response. If either the adrenals or thyroid is not functioning as it should, the other is negatively impacted.

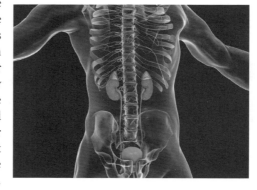

These glands belong to the endocrine system which also includes the pituitary and hypothalamus, both of which are present in the brain. Additional glands of this system include the thymus, pineal, testes, ovaries, parathyroid, and pancreas.

Adrenals

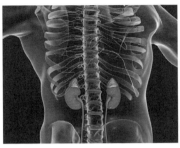

The adrenal glands sit on top of the kidneys, are triangular-shaped, and are about the size and color of a fortune cookie. They have an inner and outer region that produce hormones needed by the body. The inner region is called the cortex and from it comes hormones that control sex (androgens, estrogens), blood salt balance (aldosterone), and blood sugar balance (cortisol). The outer region, the medulla, produces the fight-or-flight hormones (collectively called adrenaline but also known as epinephrine and norepinephrine). When adrenal hormones are needed, the body sends a signal for this gland to start pumping them out.

When the adrenals are working as they should, a person wakes after a refreshing sleep with a feeling of energy. They don't *need* coffee or any other stimulant to get going; instead, they can get through all their physical and mental work for the day with only a few short breaks to eat and rest. They are able to get to sleep at night and wake rested and refreshed the next morning to do it all again because their immune, reproductive, neurological, and other systems function as they should.

When the adrenal gland is not working as it should, people often report being tired and fatigued much of the day even after a full night's sleep. They don't have enough energy and resting doesn't really help. They may also report frequent and long-lived illness, poor metabolism, blood sugar control problems, weight gain, and insomnia to name a few. An important thing to keep in mind is that the adrenals can continue to work for years, even if they are not working as well as they should before 'disease' is diagnosed. The symptoms of dysfunction can start long before the diagnosis.

Thyroid

The thyroid gland lies under the skin, in front of the esophagus across the throat. It makes hormones commonly called "thyroid hormone". The

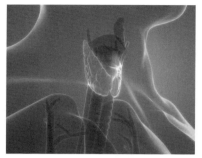

medical terms for these hormones are thyroxine (T4) and triiodothyronine (T3). Thyroid hormone controls your body's metabolism, the process in which your body transforms the food you eat into energy. Every cell of the body needs this hormone to function; without it, we die.

A properly working thyroid gland leads to sufficient energy, clear thinking, good circulation and wound healing, a better immune response, stronger muscles, and proper detoxification and elimination.

When the thyroid is not functioning properly, a chain reaction of hormonal events takes place that involves many other glands/hormones of the endocrine system and the bodily systems they regulate. The end result is one of two primary states, diagnosed as hyperthyroidism or hypothyroidism.

Hyperthyroidism results when the thyroid is overactive and more thyroid hormone is produced than the body needs. Everything in the body is on overdrive, including metabolism, frequency of bowels, emotions (anxiousness), increased sweating, and for women, very light menstruation or cessation of the menstrual cycle. A person feels hot and can't maintain a healthy weight. There are also bouts of exhaustion from the body trying to maintain this intense state of arousal.

Hypothyroidism results when the thyroid is underactive and not putting out as much thyroid hormone as needed. In this state, a person often feels tired and sluggish, gains weight, and has brittle hair and nails. One might feel cold, may be kind of depressed, or suffer from constipation. Women with this condition usually have irregular, painful, or heavy menstruation.

Working in Tandem

Like the adrenals, the thyroid can also continue to work for years before disease is diagnosed, even if it's not working as well as it should. In the case of the adrenal-thyroid system, when one is faltering, the other can take up the slack. Eventually, if health is not restored, or supported, both glands are affected and function decreases—eventually failing.

One example worth looking at involves stress hormones which will be detailed more in the next section. Cortisol, a stress hormone produced by the adrenal gland, has been linked to suppressed thyroid function which can lead to hypothyroid-like effects, especially if this stress is maintained over time. As smoking causes an increase in cortisol, this causes the thyroid gland to work harder to do its job.

Another example is adrenal fatigue. The adrenal glands can work harder in smokers versus non-smokers, and this can push the adrenals into overdrive. At some point, the glands become unable to keep up, and adrenal fatigue can set in. With elevated cortisol and adrenal levels, the thyroid signaling hormone (TSH) is suppressed. Your body thinks it is in a fight or flight situation all the time, meaning there's no time for resting and healing the body's systems. The thyroid stimulates metabolism and healing mechanisms across the body. Symptoms such as tiredness, brain fog, depression, dry skin, thinning hair, etc. can result, as both organs are negatively affected.

How Smoking Damages the Adrenal and Thyroid Systems

Smoking and how it relates to the endocrine system is a complicated affair that hasn't been nearly as well studied as systems such as the respiratory or cardiovascular. Despite this, it doesn't mean smoking doesn't impact the adrenal and thyroid glands—all parts of the body are connected, interrelated and interdependent on one another for optimal functioning. As such, it is important to understand how smoking can harm and impair the endocrine system.

Adrenals

Adrenal gland research shows that people who smoke are more likely to be tired and have less energy to get through the day. A Brazilian study found smokers moved less on a daily basis, and participants noted it was because of lower energy and a lack of motivation. Of course, in addition to the adrenal glands, smoking also affects the lungs, heart, and other organs which can also play a role in perceived energy levels.

Adrenocorticotropic hormone (*ACTH*), a substance produced in the pituitary gland is higher in smokers. ACTH acts on the adrenal glands and causes them to release cortisol and androgens (sex hormones). There are cells in the hypothalamus that are very sensitive to nicotine and when stimulated can create something called a hormone-signaling cascade. In other words, the adrenals are overproducing cortisol.

Epinephrine, more commonly known as adrenaline, and norepinephrine are two other hormones produced by the adrenals. Adrenaline is what triggers our fight-or-flight response and is supposed to only be present in bursts as needed. Both hormones have been found to be chronically higher in smokers, especially norepinephrine in the elderly. These hormones raise blood pressure and heart rate, putting smokers at a higher risk of chronic health concerns.

Smoking has been found to affect the number of steroid hormones found in the bloodstream at any one time. Research has found higher levels of the hormones DHEAS and androstenedione in smokers versus non-smokers. This may contribute, at least in part, to the insulin resistance that is reported in smokers as well as an increased risk of osteoporosis in postmenopausal smokers. After menopause, women's hormone balance is dependent on the health of the adrenal glands which take over almost all sex hormone production.

Thyroid

Smoking has a negative impact on thyroxine (T4), the thyroid's storage hormone, by causing it to be higher than the levels typically found in former or non-smokers. TSH (thyroid stimulating hormone) is lower in smokers as well. As a result, the risk of developing a thyroid autoimmune disease, such as Grave's disease or autoimmune thyroiditis, goes up.

If a smoker develops Grave's disease, they are at an even higher risk of developing eye problems such as vision disturbances and exophthalmos, otherwise described as bulging eyes. Happily, research shows these effects tend to be resolved in former smokers who have been smoke-free for six months or more.

Smoking also makes it more likely a goiter (swelling) will form in the thyroid gland. One of the reasons for this is thiocyanate, which is present in tobacco smoke. It is a chemical linked to an increased risk of developing a goiter. This is especially true in places low in iodine such as the Midwestern United States. This happens because thiocyanate slows down iodide transport into the thyroid gland as well as increases the iodide transport out of the gland, this severely compromises the thyroid's ability to have enough iodine to make thyroid hormone.

How to Support and Heal the Adrenals and Thyroid Systems

On the one hand, most body processes are strong and vibrant and hum along in the background with no conscious input. On the other hand, it requires a delicate balance and lots of cooperation between various body systems and glands for someone to feel their best. Creating basic health is the first step, and it is suggested to review Chapters 2-4 if you have not done so already.

Here are a few more, adrenal/thyroid specific strategies known to increase health in these systems.

Supplements

Both the adrenal and thyroid glands are dependent on minerals for optimal functioning. While most doctors will recommend a full-spectrum mineral, listed below are a few specific minerals which are directly related to the adrenal and thyroid glands' optimal functioning. Other minerals such as iron, copper, magnesium, molybdenum, etc., are also important, and these can be added dietarily with a multimineral or multivitamin supplement under the guidance of an experienced health practitioner.

Iodine

Humans have known iodine is critical for thyroid health for centuries. One case in point is part of the history of iodized salt in the United States. Although formally 'discovered' in 1813, iodine was used as far back as 3600 BC in China to treat goiters. By 1896, modern scientists had learned that iodine is concentrated in the thyroid gland. Goiters used to be relatively common in certain areas of the United States. These areas were often referred to as the goiter belt and included the Northwest, Midwest/Great Lakes, and Appalachian regions. Goiter was so common in Michigan that at one point it was present in up to 64% of the people living in certain areas. In order to help deal with this, iodized salt was proposed as a solution. This was a safe, relatively inexpensive, and stable way to get iodine into the population which eradicated most cases of goiter.

Using iodized salt on your foods, buying grain-based foods like bread from your local supermarket, eating dairy products, or adding in seafoods such as seaweed can help you meet your daily intake of iodine. Otherwise, multivitamins also contain iodine.

Selenium

Selenium also plays a huge role in adrenal and thyroid health. In addition to its antioxidant qualities, selenium is stored in the adrenal gland in case insufficient levels of selenium are consumed in the diet. Reduced selenium diets have been found to have a negative impact on adrenal hormone production because selenium is needed to make thyroid hormone.

Selenium is also a part of selenoproteins, a class of proteins with a wide variety of functions in the body. Most importantly for the thyroid, selenoproteins help the thyroid deal with free radicals which are produced as thyroid hormone is synthesized. If you are looking to add selenium to your diet, try Brazil nuts. They are high in selenium, and eating 2-3 daily will meet and exceed the daily recommended intake.

Zinc

Zinc has been found to have a direct relationship with adrenal and thyroid hormones. In general, this mineral is responsible for over 300 chemical reactions in the body. In animal studies done more than 20 years ago, zinc was found to play an important role in the function of thyroid receptors and in producing hormone carrier proteins. Interestingly, the relationship with the body's ability to absorb zinc is also related to the amount of thyroid hormone in the body. In deficient or hypothyroid states, there is less zinc present; in excess or hyperthyroid states, zinc is abundant.

You can get a zinc supplement of 20-30 mg in the form of zinc citrate or zinc picolinate which are more bioavailable forms. If you prefer food sources, oysters, red meat, chicken, beans, nuts, whole grain foods, and dairy products contain zinc. Because zinc can interfere with iron and copper absorption, please note it is not recommended to supplement this regularly for more than three months without checking in with your doctor.

More information about minerals can be found in Chapters 3 and 4 specifically and is discussed throughout most chapters of this book.

Glandulars

Glandulars are supplements made from animal glandular material, otherwise known as organotherapy, and have been used to support human health and wellness for practically as long as health records have been kept. Organotherapy can be used for any glandular organ in the body, although here the focus is on the thyroid and adrenal glands.

There are several ways in which glandular supplements are made, but it is recommended to use a company that freeze-dries their animal material. This keeps all of the essential elements including nutrients and hormones intact. For best results and reduced possibility of contamination, the animals should be grass-fed in pesticide-free fields and as hormone-free as possible. Most glandulars will contain fatty cellular material from the animals, and as fat holds onto contaminants, this makes sourcing glandulars from high-quality material imperative. Dosing with glandulars varies greatly on the type of glandular supplement.

Glandulars are a safe therapy with relatively little risk, especially when high-quality source animals are used. Cows and pigs are most commonly used, although sheep and other animals can be used. Bovine spongiform encephalopathy, more commonly known as mad cow disease, is potentially possible if glandular material is extracted from infected cattle. Again, just make sure you are getting glandulars from a reputable source. As always, visit your holistic health practitioner to learn if this therapy may be helpful for you.

Vitamin B Complex

As mentioned previously, cigarette smoking causes excess cortisol production from the adrenal gland. One way to help counteract some of this damage is by supplementing with B complex. Research has shown B vitamins, especially B6 (pyridoxine), B9 (folate), and B12 (cobalamin) act to lower stress and relieve tiredness. A double-blind placebo controlled trial of 138 adults found, after 16 weeks of taking a multivitamin with B vitamins, salivary cortisol levels were lower. For more information about B vitamins, see Chapters 4, 8, 11, 14, and 17-18.

Botanicals

Ashwagandha

Ashwagandha (*Withania somnifera*) is an adaptogenic herb that has been used for centuries in Ayurvedic and Chinese medical applications. It's an evergreen shrub most commonly seen in India, the Middle East, and Africa. It has been shown to be a potent antioxidant. It is also anti-inflammatory, blood-supporting, neuroprotective, supports and expands memory capabilities, increases sleep health, and can help with anxious moods.

Research indicates this can lower cortisol which has been shown to be higher in smokers, especially those smoking ten or more cigarettes daily.

Ashwagandha also helps improve sleep quality, helps with anxiety, eating behaviors, and mental wellness in overweight or obese adults.

The common dosing recommendation is at least 2 grams daily in divided doses. Remember that herbs work best when they are taken regularly each day. Adaptogenic herbs are slower, deeper acting plants, so taking them for at least three months will help you achieve the best result possible.

Holy Basil

Holy Basil (*Ocimum sanctum*), also known as tulsi or tulasi, is another plant with deep historical roots in treating human health concerns over hundreds of years. Its importance to Indian culture has been solidified with its medical applications as well as its spiritual applications in sacred rituals. Holy Basil is an adaptogenic herb that has a variety of health-supporting aspects including antimicrobial and anti-inflammatory actions, as well as being protective of the liver, brain, and cardiovascular system.

It can help support the body with stress, minimizing toxins and damage caused by radiation exposure, and can also help with blood sugar dysregulation.

Animal studies have demonstrated that Holy Basil contains compounds that increase stress tolerance and support a healthy adrenal gland, especially when administered before a stress-inducing situation. It has also been found to lift low spirits and a depressed mood, help with drug and nicotine withdrawal, and was found to be protective of smoke-induced lung damage.

You can use whole herb tinctures and extracts or take Holy Basil as a tea.

Licorice

Licorice (*Glycyrrhiza glabra*) has been used for thousands of years with the earliest known example found in ancient Egyptian pharaoh's tombs including King Tut's. It was also documented on Assyrian records in 2,000 or 3,000 BCE. It was used historically for a multitude of health concerns such as in the treatment of asthma, as a cold tonic, in support of healthy blood sugars, and was also used to help postpone hunger and thirst.

One of licorice's actions is to inhibit the breakdown of cortisol in the body, allowing it to remain in the bloodstream longer. This gives the adrenal glands, producers of cortisol, support especially under chronic stress conditions.

In general, it is not recommended to use this herb regularly in large doses for long periods of time without guidance from a qualified practitioner. This herb is not recommended for use in those who are pregnant, nursing, or have high blood pressure without first consulting their doctor or a qualified holistic health practitioner. In people who tend to have swelling due to salt intake, this herb should be avoided completely.

Lemon Balm

Lemon balm (*Melissa officinalis*) should be mentioned for stress management. It is an easy-to-grow perennial that is tolerant of growing conditions in a wide variety of environments. Herbalists sometimes refer to it as "sunshine-in-a-plant", meaning it can provide a lightening of mood for an individual in a more anxious or depressive state due to its mild nervine action. It is also an antiviral, antibacterial, antifungal, and antioxidant herb which can also have a pain-modulating effect. Additionally, it is supportive of the cardiovascular system due to its effects on cholesterol and its potential capacity for modulating heart rates in a recent animal study. Though more research needs to be conducted before results can be considered definitive.

This herb is easy to incorporate into your daily routine, especially if you can make space to grow this in a pot or your garden. Once you grow it, you can dry it towards the end of the season, giving yourself a supply of home-grown tea through the winter months.

Lifestyle

Diet

It is always recommended to practice a balanced healthy diet, as there can be benefits from including/excluding certain things. As always, making sure you have adequate minerals in your diet is important, but in this system specifically, certain minerals are needed for your organs to work properly. Some of these minerals have been mentioned previously in the supplements section such as selenium, iodine, and zinc. In addition, a good multimineral is also supportive in stressful situations. Make sure your minerals include magnesium and calcium as well since both can help promote relaxation mentally and physically.

The foods you may need vary depending on if your thyroid is hypofunctioning or hyperfunctioning. Minerals are good no matter what condition your thyroid is in. In addition to being found in Brazil nuts, selenium can be found in other foods such as eggs, tuna, sardines, and legumes. Zinc can be found in shellfish such as oysters, beef, and chicken. In cases of hypothyroidism, foods which can be supportive include seaweeds, fish, dairy, and eggs as they are a natural source of iodine.

In cases of hyperthyroidism, avoiding high-iodine foods is essential. Adding non-iodized salt, egg whites, canned or fresh fruit, oats, potatoes, honey, maple syrup, etc., can help with this. It is also recommended to eat goitrogenic foods. These are foods that can interfere with thyroid function. People with hypothyroid are usually cautioned to avoid goitrogens. Foods in this category include cruciferous vegetables like broccoli, bok choy, cabbage, spinach, kale, etc. Others are soy foods like tempeh and tofu, sweet potatoes, cassava, peaches, strawberries, and finally some nuts and seeds including peanuts and pine nuts. Millet, especially pearl millet, is considered a goitrogen and appears to affect the thyroid whether a person is an overall healthy individual or mineral deficient (iodine and/or selenium).

Research is still ongoing to determine how many cruciferous vegetables at one time or how many weekly servings can cause this effect. Overall, goitrogens are not a huge issue via labs for thyroid health, but it's important to rotate the foods you eat daily and as always, you need to consume all foods in moderation. It is definitely possible to have too much of a good thing.

Last but not least, there are foods that can be supportive of adrenal function. It is most important to eat regular meals to maintain a good blood sugar level throughout the day. In cases of adrenal fatigue, it's important to eat as few processed foods as possible, especially synthetic sweeteners, fried foods, and soft drinks. Try your best to eat whole foods with minimal processing. Your plate should be roughly half vegetables with a small amount of low-sugar fruit, roughly ¼ to ⅓ protein, and the rest can be healthy fats such as avocado or olive oil and whole grains. Proteins can include lean meats, legumes, fish, dairy, or nuts. Turmeric, black pepper, and green chilies are spices which may help balance out thyroid function. As always, assuming your digestive tract is working well and absorbing nutrients properly, getting nutrients from foods prevents overdosing which can be possible if you are taking supplements without medical guidance.

While the diet is discussed in numerous chapters of this book, an in-depth discussion can be found in Chapters 3 and 4.

Exercise

Exercise is important for thyroid health whether you have hypo- or hyperthyroid symptoms. If things in your body are sluggish, movement can help speed things up and make weight management easier to deal with. In the case of things working at an accelerated pace, exercise can help with anxiety, fatigue, or sleep problems. Any way you can increase movement daily is a strong way to improve your overall health. More information about exercise can be found in Chapter 3.

- Yoga

    There are specific poses in yoga that can be used to stimulate proper thyroid functioning. Small studies have supported this claim though more research is needed. It's important to note descriptions of the poses themselves are a bit more complex and beyond the scope of this book. Consider finding a good yoga teacher, though you may be able to find some of these specific poses in online videos which can help guide you. A few specific poses include the supported shoulder stand, plow pose, fish pose, legs-up-the-wall pose, or cat-cow pose. Other options may be available under the guidance of a trained yoga instructor.

- Resistance Training

    This type of training appears to have a significant positive impact on thyroid hormone levels. Research has found an hour a day of regular exercise over the course of three months causes significant changes in regulating hormone levels in hypothyroid males. More research is needed in this area, especially with most research being done on healthy males.

    Resistance training can be done at the gym by yourself or with help from an experienced trainer who can show you the proper form for the exercises. If you've never used light weights or bands before, having someone show you how to use them properly may be the best way to add resistance training into your routine. There are also online videos that can explain a few of these exercises. Remember this doesn't have to be done daily for any positive effect. At a minimum, it's recommended to exercise for 30 minutes three times a week. Gentle exercises or resistance training a few days a week can have a positive impact on thyroid and adrenal health.

Social Support

Lack of community is often a central theme for people who experience thyroid and adrenal dysfunction. A common suggestion from holistic practitioners is to make time for social support. The following are a few ideas you can use to help find a group of like-minded folks.

- Shared Interest Groups

    You can check out Meetup.com or find local groups on social media that share your interests. Rock climbing or collecting? Fossil hunting? Hiking or cooking? Find others who like to do what you do and go hang out with them.

- Trauma Support Groups

    As this is another common underlying cause of adrenal and thyroid issues, this could be a powerful tool in your healing journey.

- Spiritual or Religious Groups

    Human beings have come together for millennia for celebration and worship in many different forms. This may be something for you to consider no matter what your beliefs may be.

Other Therapies to Consider

Stress Management

This includes any and all tools which help you manage your stress. If you don't have any stress management tools that you've utilized in the past, it's easy to start learning new ways to help. Most importantly, you have to carve personal time out for yourself every week in order to accomplish this. If you are a busy young professional, married or single with children, a business owner, etc., there is always a list of things to accomplish, and it's important to realize the list will never end. Taking time out for yourself can be 30 minutes a day to read or exercise, an afternoon to go on a hike or visit a new place, or taking an entire weekend to yourself once or twice a month where you just shut off your phone and computer. Each of these scenarios are ways you can use small lifestyle tools to manage your stress. Additional suggestions include watching a movie, going for a daily walk in a natural setting, doing hobbies such as sewing or playing an instrument, or some other activity you find relaxing. If you have trouble figuring this out for yourself, you can find a life coach who can help put stress management tools into a perspective that works well for you.

Counseling

Past or more recent traumas can have an impact on overall health. Many times an imbalance in a person's emotional state first shows up in decreased adrenal and thyroid function. You can talk to your doctor or local health practitioner for referrals for various types of counselors depending on your individual needs and preferences.

Chapter 13:
Keeping Your Metabolism on Track

One of the most common things people report when they try to quit smoking is weight gain. In fact, it is not uncommon for people to keep smoking as a weight control measure. People indeed seem to gain weight after they quit smoking, but the effects of smoking on the metabolic system are more far-reaching than just a number on the scale. Nicotine revs up the system; it increases heart rate, alters blood sugar chemistry, affects lipid (fat) chemistry, and activates the sympathetic nervous system (flight/fight).

There are things you can do to create a healthier metabolism, although many of the negative effects cannot be altered as long as the chemicals from what you are smoking are circulating in your body. In the meantime, let's focus on what you can do!

The Metabolic System

The metabolic system is not so much a system as it is a collection of chemical reactions taking place within each cell of the body. It can be as complex as you want it to be. It may be helpful to think of it as one large system, including the whole human body, and understand it as:

1. The breaking down and absorption of nutrients
2. The building of a new body using those nutrients

In step one, the nutrients are converted into energy and in step two, the body uses that energy to rebuild. Scientists who study the metabolic system call this catabolism (breaking down) and anabolism (building up).

The metabolic system includes your entire body. To understand this better, a few terms are useful to understand.

- Calorie

    A calorie is defined as the energy needed to raise the temperature of 1 gram of water through 1 °C (now usually defined as 4.19 joules). A calorie is a unit of measure for the energy that comes from certain foods. For example, water has no caloric intake, whereas a chocolate milkshake can have 450 or more calories.

- Basal Metabolic Rate (BMR)

    BMR is commonly referred to as your resting metabolic rate (RMR); it is the number of calories needed by your body to sustain life. This accounts for roughly 70% of the calories you intake. Another 20% is needed for physical activity, and the last 10% is the energy needed for digestion to break down your food. It's important to keep in mind a lot of factors play a role in determining how many calories a person might need including mineral deficiencies, body weight (larger versus slimmer body structure), age, growth (children burn more than adults while they are growing), hormones, and even gender. There are calculators online that you can use to determine this, and you can download apps on your smart devices to help track your daily caloric intake.

So, what does all that mean for a smoker? Nicotine acts on the human metabolic system like fuel to a fire, making the system work faster and more furiously. As the average American gets too little movement on a daily basis and tends to eat too many calories for what their body needs to function, one of nicotine's many effects is that some people find it easier to control their weight. Some smokers originally start because of this, and others refuse to quit because of the fear of weight gain. In most cases, nicotine withdrawal itself isn't causing weight gain, but rather the increase in high-calorie comfort foods which commonly follows smoking cessation.

How Smoking Damages Your Metabolism

In addition to nicotine raising BMR, it can also cause other damaging effects. As discussed in Chapter 12, smoking has an effect on the adrenal gland causing an increase in adrenaline, this explains how nicotine revs up the system. Over time, smoking causes the adrenal gland to work at a high capacity for too long which leads to some of the health concerns previously discussed. The more you smoke, the worse this effect can be.

Metabolic syndrome, which was previously mentioned in relation to reproductive health, should be mentioned again. This syndrome is a set of health parameters that, when outside normal ranges, dramatically increases the risk of coronary disease, heart attack, stroke, diabetes, and a laundry list of other serious health conditions. Metabolic syndrome is common in the average American with an estimated one in three adults having it.

Smokers are at an increased risk for metabolic syndrome. Nicotine usage helps cover up some of the weight gain difficulties which can occur but can elevate other metrics of metabolic syndrome including high blood pressure, high "bad cholesterol" (LDL), low "good cholesterol" (HDL), and high blood sugars. Smoking has repeatedly been linked with the accumulation of abdominal fat and insulin resistance (meaning the body has a harder time dealing with glucose from food). Heavier smokers generally gain the most weight, overcoming nicotine's weight-loss effect. Even years after smoking cessation the increased risk for metabolic syndrome can remain.

How to Support and Heal Metabolism

Because a person's metabolism involves the entire body, it is difficult to say if there are things that truly heal metabolism. Instead, focus on elevating the overall health of your body with proper diet, hydration, sleep, exercise, and detoxification. Because blood sugar control and weight management are two areas many smokers struggle with, the suggestions in this book focus on things that can help with weight.

Supplements

Psyllium Husk

Psyllium husk (*Plantago ovata*) is a plant that now grows in Europe and across Asia but was originally thought to have come from central Asia. In the modern era, almost all psyllium husk is grown in India. There, in addition to health support, it is used as animal feed, to prevent slipping on ice, and as a food additive. Primarily, it has been used as an anti-diarrheal, a laxative, and to help prevent vomiting.

A high-fiber diet can help reduce metabolic syndrome. The seed of psyllium husk is probably best known as a good source of fiber to help prevent constipation. What sets it apart from a few other fiber-rich plants is its slimy texture when the seeds or powder are mixed with water. Overall, research has shown success in lowering blood pressure and supporting healthy cholesterol levels. It has also been reported to help lower appetite levels which can be helpful for former smokers managing their weight.

As most smokers tend to not make healthy diet choices, adding in psyllium husk can be helpful. For more information about fiber, see Chapters 3, 8, 12, and 16.

Inositol

Inositol is a type of sugar, otherwise known as a carbohydrate, present in supplements and foods. The body even produces it inside the cells. There are several inositols, myoinositol being the most prevalent. Inositols in general are secondary messengers which allow the cells to communicate, and they are also part of the cells' membrane, allowing it to respond to external messages such as hormones and neurotransmitters. It is also directly involved with reproductive health in men and women. Inositol has been used previously for panic disorder, depression, obsessive-compulsive disorder, and polycystic ovarian disorder (PCOS) with varying degrees of success.

In addition to being researched for lots of other health concerns, inositol has been looked at recently for its effect on non-alcoholic fatty liver disease (NAFLD). NAFLD is now considered the liver aspect of metabolic syndrome due to its causative features. Animal studies have shown in creatures with NAFLD, the liver is deficient in inositol, and when those animals were supplemented, they had reduced liver triglycerides and cholesterol. Inositol also lowered liver enzymes and helped to preserve vitamins E and C stores in the liver and has been shown to help improve insulin resistance, though the exact mechanism is unknown at this time.

If you prefer to get Inositol from your diet, bran, seeds, beans, and peas are among the richest sources as well as melon and citrus. Otherwise, supplementation has been shown to be safe in high doses of up to several grams daily.

Chromium

Chromium is a mineral that is common in two forms. One is trivalent chromium which is essential in trace amounts to human health, and the other is hexavalent which is toxic. Chromium is important to food metabolism as it helps insulin function more efficiently. It allows the body to use less insulin to achieve desired blood sugar levels.

You can get chromium from your diet, but levels vary widely depending on the region where your food was grown and how the food was processed. One reference noted a fifty-fold difference in chromium levels in oatmeal alone. A few foods which may be higher in chromium include grape juice, ham, brewer's yeast, beef, orange juice, and turkey breast. Additionally, eating fewer simple sugars in your diet and keeping stress levels under control helps preserve chromium in the body.

For supplementation, taking minerals with food for improved absorption is recommended. Chromium picolinate is one of the best and most widely used forms of chromium and can be supplemented at 200 mcg once or twice daily. Please note that some multivitamins contain chromium so you may already be getting some on a daily basis without even realizing it! For more information about chromium, see Chapters 4 and 7.

Botanicals

Artichoke

Artichoke (*Cynara cardunculus var. scolymus*) has a rich history with its earliest recorded beginning in Ancient Greece and Rome where it was popularly used as both a food and medicine. Its image was also found on ancient Egyptian tablets and altars. Nowadays, it is still a common staple in the Mediterranean diet. It contains Vitamin C, minerals, and fiber. Artichoke is an antioxidant, antimicrobial, liver protective, and helps reduce cholesterol levels. Artichoke has also been found to support healthy blood sugar levels. Because of this, artichoke is primarily used to support the gallbladder and liver, both of which are very important for a healthy metabolism.

Modern science has demonstrated artichoke can help lower LDL cholesterol and raise HDL, reducing the risk of future heart disease. Additionally, it has been shown to help reduce atherosclerotic plaques, a buildup of cholesterol in the blood vessels which increases the risk of heart attacks. Research has shown it has the potential to help increase bile excretion, and it is also protective of the liver itself though the exact mechanisms are still being researched at this time.

Artichoke can be taken once a day long term to help support liver health, and it is generally well-tolerated. If you are on blood pressure medication or diabetic medications, please talk with your doctor before using this herb.

Milk Thistle

As mentioned previously in Chapter 8, milk thistle (*Silybum marianum*) can be a way to aid the metabolic system. In addition to being liver supportive and protective, it can help lower blood sugar levels by supporting beta cells in the pancreas which are responsible for making and secreting insulin. Milk thistle also helps lower cholesterol levels. In patients with cirrhosis and diabetes, taking milk thistle daily lowered their HbA1c by an average of 0.5% and decreased insulin requirements by up to 20% per day.

Milk thistle is best taken in whole herb form as capsules with a milk thistle extract concentration of at least 70% silybin. It is safe at higher doses but research has shown support for dosing 240 mg - 900 mg two to three times a day. If you are currently taking diabetic medications, consult your doctor before taking milk thistle.

Lifestyle

Diet

As always, diet is one of the foundational pieces to overall health. For more in-depth information on the aspects of a well-balanced, whole-foods diet, please reference Chapters 3 and 4. Many of my smoking patients have found great success with an insulin resistance diet. The core plan is to focus on including foods that have the least amount of processing possible. Below are some dietary suggestions to guide you.

- No Whites Diet

    One simple step you can use to start incorporating a more healthy diet is by avoiding foods that are white. These foods tend to be more highly processed and/or less nutrient dense than other food options. There are healthier, more nutrient-dense white foods out there, so just avoid white foods which are more sugar/carbohydrate-dense, and less vitamin and mineral dense. One example is choosing a sweet potato or parsnip instead of a white potato. White rice, white flour, white bread, white sugar, white pasta, white potatoes/potato chips, salt, etc., are all included on this list. Remember, this is much less about dieting versus moving to create a healthier lifestyle for yourself and your family.

- Low Glycemic Foods

    This is a system that was developed, ranking foods from 1 to 100 based on how large of an impact that particular food has on blood sugar levels. This is determined by having 10 healthy people eat 50 grams of carbohydrates of the food and monitoring their blood sugar levels for the next two hours. Their results are compared to 10 healthy people consuming 50 grams of glucose/sugar. Low glycemic foods are ranked 55 or less, moderate glycemic foods are 56 - 69, and high glycemic foods are 70 or higher.

    In general, for those who have weight/cholesterol issues, cardiovascular health concerns, or are diabetic, eating a majority of their diet as low glycemic index foods can help with their overall health and wellness. In smokers, whose bodies are already working overtime dealing with extra toxin load and higher risk of metabolic syndrome, this can be helpful. For more information on specific foods, you can reference https://glycemicindex.com.

Exercise

As always, exercise has a major impact on overall health. Exercise has been shown to reduce weight, improve cholesterol profiles, and increase insulin sensitivity. Research shows up to a 58% reduction in the risk of developing diabetes in populations who made lifestyle changes including exercise. Another study looked at healthy but sedentary adults, and after 20 weeks of using an exercise bike 3 times a week, 30% of those who had metabolic syndrome were no longer diagnosable with it. Adding in more movement than what you are currently doing is key. You can learn more about exercise in Chapters 3, 7, 11, and 12.

Other Therapies to Consider

Hydrotherapy

As the metabolic system touches on every major system in the body, it's important to work from a whole-body perspective. Hydrotherapy is very supportive of overall health and well-being. The most often type of hydrotherapy suggested is constitutional hydrotherapy as it works to increase circulation to the entire body. As you improve your diet, add in some more movement, and potentially some herbal support, constitutional hydrotherapy will help these tools to be more effective. You can find instructions for a home version of this therapy in the Apothecary section or find a practitioner that offers this service in office. More information about hydrotherapy can be found in Chapter 4.

Chapter 14:
The Mental and Emotional You

Every time you finish a cigarette, your body starts to clean up the mess. Nicotine and other chemical levels drop as your body starts to detox and repair tissue; next, you start to experience withdrawal. You will often see symptoms like a cough, acute hearing or taste, sweating, anxiety, or hunger. In addition to physical symptoms, people often experience emotional swings such as feeling weepy, angry, sad, and irritable. Mental states can also become disordered, and result in restlessness, anxiety, and difficulty concentrating. These mental and emotional states can shift rapidly and in extreme ways. People often describe themselves as irrational until they get their smoke. This is withdrawal.

While each person is affected differently and to varying levels by nicotine and other chemicals, everyone experiences withdrawal symptoms to some degree. How long someone can go without their next smoke also varies. The average amount of time it takes to experience withdrawal symptoms ranges from 4 - 24 hours. But, withdrawal can happen as quickly as 10 minutes after you put that smoke out, especially the emotional symptoms. Maybe this is one reason why some people chain-smoke. For people who quit, physical withdrawal symptoms usually pass after a couple of weeks while emotional and mental disorder can take much longer.

Often smokers feel when their mental and emotional state is disturbed they need a cigarette. They are convinced, by lighting up, things will level off and they will be able to function again. As it turns out, this sense of being helped by having a smoke is a trick. Smokers do feel an immediate sensation of relaxation, but they aren't really any better.

It's important to realize there's a strong association between smoking and mental health problems. Those diagnosed with mental illness have a higher rate of smoking than those who aren't diagnosed with a psychiatric concern. Those who have multiple disorders including schizophrenia, mood, anxiety, eating, and/or addictive disorders are 2-5 times more likely to be smokers. Research reveals that smoking increases anxiety, depression, and stress, all while lowering overall positive regard for life. Smoking also creates sleeping problems and is strongly correlated to an increased risk of suicide. It's important to realize the positive feeling smokers have when they light one is made possible by dopamine, which functions as a neurotransmitter in the brain. With smoking, the brain is rewarded through dopamine by feeling good after inhaling, but this is just a temporary shift in biochemistry.

How Smoking Damages the Mental and Emotional You

Smoking is hard on your body in many ways and this includes your physical brain, how well it works in a variety of capacities, and, perhaps most importantly, how it affects your emotions. Modern science has linked smoking to depression, dysthymia, panic and social anxiety disorders, post-traumatic stress disorder (PTSD), and generalized anxiety disorder (GAD). The more you smoke, the more your mental and emotional states are negatively impacted. If you slow down or stop smoking, this effect decreases, especially over time as your body heals.

Research supports a strong association between smoking and several psychiatric disorders including ADHD and an increased risk of developing dementia/Alzheimer's Disease. Studies are also actively looking at the risk factors between smoking and bipolar disorder as well as the development and perpetuation of anxiety disorders. While it's true using nicotine seems to improve cognition, memory, and attention in healthy individuals, for chronic smokers, it results in cognitive declines, especially with remembering words and the speed of processing thoughts in middle-aged to elderly smokers.

Physical brain degeneration has also been found with imaging, and it's not limited by age. Decreased gray matter in the brain has been visualized in smokers' brains who are under 30 years of age. Gray matter is the collection of neurons in the brain responsible for its ability to function. White matter, the myelinated connections between neurons that allows them to communicate more effectively, has been found to break down more as the years someone smokes accumulate. Overall, this means brain mass shrinks with smoking, and it is worse in those who smoke more cigarettes per day and in those who have been smoking for years.

Additionally, smoking is also associated with sleep disturbances. Nicotine use seems to make it harder to fall asleep as well as wake up in the morning, potentially due to nicotine's stimulating effects. Women were also found to be more sleepy during the day, and men were found to have more disturbing dreams or nightmares. There is also a link between smoking and suicide. Both current and former smokers appear to have an increased risk of suicide. The exact reason is still being studied, but with all the negative effects smoking can have on the body, this isn't necessarily surprising.

How to Support and Heal the Mental and Emotional You

Research has made it very clear, the healthier the state of your body, the better you feel, and the more resilient and balanced you are. Smoking introduces a constant stream of toxins into your body and, in addition to maintaining basic good health, there are specific things that may help you increase your overall level of health. If you have not already, this is a great opportunity to review Chapters 2-4 once again. In addition to the basics, when it comes to the brain and your mental and emotional state, the following may be helpful.

Supplements

Trace Minerals

Trace minerals are critical to overall health. These minerals, including selenium, zinc, and copper have consistently been shown to be essential for your mental well-being. As tobacco smoke uses up the body's resources faster, trace minerals become all the more important. As mentioned in Chapters 3 and 4, minerals play a huge role in detoxification.

EFAs

Essential Fatty Acids (EFAs), commonly found in fish oil, are critical to health in smokers due to their antioxidant and anti-inflammatory abilities. The body cannot make these fats, so folks have to supplement them in their diet or use nutritional products. One study in 2014 found supplementing with EFAs lowered the number of cigarettes used and tobacco cravings. Study participants took over two grams each of EPA and DHA on a daily basis for one month. Even after the study ended, tobacco cravings were still reduced the following month. EFA imbalances affect dopamine and this may contribute to the raised frequency of cravings. For more information about EFAs, see Chapters 4, 7, 9-10, 15, 17, and 19.

Probiotics

Studies show probiotics can have a positive effect on depression and depressed mood. Researchers analyzed effects on mood, anxiety, and cognition and found positive results on all measures of depressive symptoms. The strain of probiotics, dosing, and duration of treatment varied widely. Scientists are also looking at gut health and its relationship to Alzheimer's Disease.

Promising studies have demonstrated probiotics may help reduce cognitive decline. Since some species of microorganisms are anti-inflammatory, antioxidant, and help lower neuroinflammation, it is easy to see how this may be helpful and supportive in smokers. For more information about probiotics, see Chapters 4, 15-16, and 19.

Botanicals

Green Oat

Oat (*Avena sativa*) research has shown even a single dose of green oat can improve cognitive function. When over one gram of green oat is taken daily for a month, it not only helps improve cognitive function but also increases physical stress tolerance. It has also been shown to be helpful with depression, providing a tonic effect on the brain and mind by supporting neurotransmitters. A small study found taking an oat tincture daily lowered cigarette cravings, which is great news for current smokers. For more information about oat, see Chapters 10, 15, and 18.

Green Tea

Green tea (*Camellia sinensis*) has been used in human societies culturally and medicinally for centuries. It was discovered by accident when a dead tea leaf was boiled and drunk by Emperor Shennong in 2737 BC. Green tea was expensive and a precious commodity for many centuries after its finding, but eventually it made its way into European markets.

Green tea has been found to have acute effects on the brain. Research indicates it has a relaxing effect by modulating stress, and along with the caffeine it contains, green tea can help people feel more alert with less mental tiredness. In those over age 55, several studies found green tea enhanced memory, information processing, and decision-making abilities when consumed daily. It has also been found to lower the risk of dementia and can even potentially help increase creativity as well as work performance.

Green tea is generally recognized as safe and can be consumed as a supplement or a tea. Since tea increases your daily water intake, adding this into your routine can be a great option. Drinking one cup of green tea daily is best to maximize its ability to protect memory and other cognitive functions.

Lifestyle

Diet

As always, it's important to maintain a healthy diet. You can refer back to Chapters 3 and 4 to remind yourself how to incorporate a whole food, less processed, diet into your daily life. Keep in mind there are professionals out there who can help you fine-tune your diet if you would like additional support. Nutritional counselors or registered dietitians can work with you to make sure you are getting the proper blend of vitamins, minerals, and other nutrients in your diet.

Exercise

Exercise helps the body release endorphins. Rather than suggesting specific exercises here, it is more important to stress the importance of moving your body. For more information on exercise and how to incorporate it into your daily/weekly routine please refer to the exercise section of Chapters 7, 11, 12, and 13.

Other Therapies to Consider

Deep Breathing Practice

You've probably heard it's good to take a deep breath every once in a while, but did you know simply breathing can relieve stress? Deep breathing techniques have been found to activate the parasympathetic system, promoting relaxation and calm while also deactivating the sympathetic fight-or-flight system. Science supports this. Diaphragmatic breathing lowers cortisol, one of our primary stress hormones. Additionally, deep breathing can increase alertness, focus, and overall comfort while reducing anxiety, depression, anger, and confusion.

Deep belly breathing was reviewed in Chapter 6. Another way to incorporate deep breathing is through guided meditations which focus on breath and relaxing the body, one part at a time. There are also guided online videos you can watch as well as downloadable apps to help you track your breathing.

Grounding

Grounding, also called earthing, is a therapeutic technique based on the laws of physics. In physics, grounding, also called earthing, provides a path for current to flow into the ground and excess electric charge to disperse instead of building up. In the context of using this as a therapy, grounding allows the excess charge in the body to disperse into the earth. To ground the body, one stays in sustained contact with the ground using their bare feet or hands. In countries where most people wear shoes throughout the day, it's interesting to find the benefit of going without them. Health benefits from releasing excess charge include increased wound healing, stress relief, a more positive mood, and decreased inflammation in the body.

This can be done in many different ways. You can simply lay on the ground or walk around your yard barefoot. If you are unable to make it outside, grounding equipment is available for purchase. Grounding devices include mats, sheets or blankets, socks, and patches or bands that you can wear throughout the day.

Chapter 15:
The Smoldering Nerves

The nervous system is like an electrical superhighway in constant motion. Little electrical signals are traveling at rapid speeds throughout your entire system lighting up nerves all over the body with information.

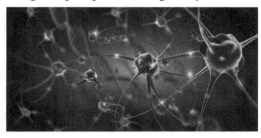

In order for this system to work at its best it must be able to move those electrical signals in a smooth, un-interrupted way. The signals travel along the nervous system but they also talk to other parts of your body, like your muscles and organs along the way. This means the membranes of all your body's cells must be intact and healthy. Smoking introduces a number of chemicals into the body that can have a negative effect on this system. Before you can consider the ways to support your nervous system you need to know more about it.

The Nervous System

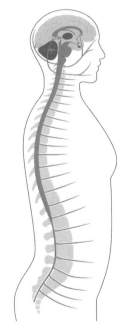

The nervous system is one of the most complex systems in your body and it interacts with every other system. There are two main parts to the nervous system. The central nervous system includes the brain and the spinal cord.

The brain consists of two hemispheres commonly referred to as the right and left hemispheres. They are connected by a structure called the corpus callosum. The brain is responsible for all higher-level thought which includes making memories, moving, feeling things physically and emotionally, etc. The rest of the central nervous system includes the spinal cord which innervates the rest of the body via spinal nerves. The cerebellum, the twisty worm-like structure on the back of the brain, is used for coordination and balance. The brainstem connects

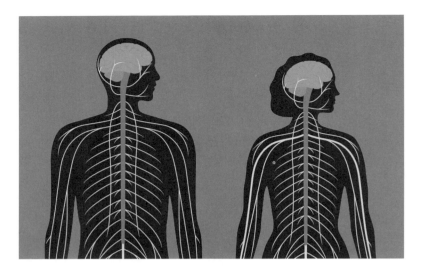

the brain to the spinal cord and is responsible for basic body functions including breathing, heartbeat regulation, eating, and sleeping.

The peripheral nervous system includes all the nerves outside of the central nervous system. These nerves help your brain send and receive messages from the other structures in your body. Part of this system is the autonomic nervous system which includes the parasympathetic "rest and digest" and sympathetic "fight or flight" system motor nerves that cause muscles, glands, and organs to function. This system also includes the sensory nerves which relay information from the world to the brain. Altogether, these two parts, the peripheral and central nervous system, communicate with each other and the rest of the body. This communication network is critical to overall health and well-being.

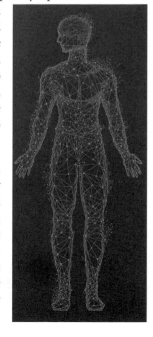

When the nervous system is working as it should, a person knows when in time they are, where they are, if they are safe, in pain, and if they should move or stop. They know when they are hungry, tired, cold, or hot. They know how hard to grasp something and how hard to throw something. They can think clearly and remember things from one minute to the next—that is, except for the location of their car keys! They can learn new things and teach things to others. They are also calm, patient, and generally in a good mood. All of this is possible because of a well-functioning nervous system.

The nervous system touches and interacts with your entire body, when it is not working as it should there can be many different kinds of symptoms. Physical symptoms like pain or numbness, burning, tingling, and fatigue can manifest as well as symptoms like anxiety, depression, fluctuating emotions, and poor cognitive function.

How Smoking Damages the Nervous System

Smoking introduces a number of chemicals into the body which can have a negative effect on this system. The blood-brain barrier (BBB) is affected by the toxins and oxidative elements of cigarette smoke. The BBB is what protects our brains from many toxins and chemicals encountered on a daily basis. Smoking is directly correlated with a loosening in the junction of these cells, allowing more substances to get through between the cells than would normally be allowed. Additionally, smoking increases inflammation which further compromises the BBB's integrity.

Smoking also increases the risk of developing neuropathic pain. The longer and more you smoke, the higher the risk, and if the smoker has any other diseases such as diabetes, the risk is even higher. Cigarette usage also causes damage to the nerves themselves. One study looked at 40 healthy smokers and 40 healthy non-smokers and found that sensory nerves in smokers reacted more slowly. The speed at which the nerve impulses slowed was directly related to how much that person smoked.

Additionally, there's a link between ulnar nerve entrapment and smoking. Ulnar nerve entrapment is when your ulnar nerve, running from your neck down into your hands, becomes pinched and causes pain and muscle weakness in the forearm and hand. Researchers found, again, the more and longer the smoker uses cigarettes, the higher the risk of developing this condition. These two major findings led the authors of the study to encourage refraining from smoking while nerve injuries heal.

Keep in mind that smoking affects all parts of the body. Also, remember that all the systems of the body affect one another. When one is struggling, such as the cardiovascular system, everything else is affected as well. The nervous system touches every single part of the body which in turn relies on receiving and sending information to function optimally. If the nerves are struggling, so is everything else.

How to Support and Heal the Nervous System

In the case of smokers, every single smoke introduces poisons into the body and affects all systems, including the nerve network and brain. Your primary job, for as long as you smoke, is to support your body and assist its healing attempts. Luckily some things can be done, taken, and eaten to help with the daily damage from smoking.

Supplements

Before continuing please refer to the supplements introduced in Chapter 4, as they will help with understanding the information in this section.

B Vitamins

Smokers tend to have lower levels of B vitamins in their system. Newer research suggests B12 is present in smokers at comparable levels to that of non-smokers, but it is an inactive form the body isn't able to utilize as effectively. The nerves rely on B vitamins, especially B1, B6, and B12 for overall nerve health and to repair nerves from injury. This makes supplementing B vitamins in the smoking population even more important. For more information about B vitamins, see Chapters 4, 8, 11-12, 14, and 17.

Magnesium

Remember, magnesium is responsible for over 300 chemical reactions in the body. Part of those reactions include supporting the nervous system for nerve transmission and for making the muscles respond to those nerve signals. A lack of magnesium increases the risk of developing neurological disorders such as migraines, chronic pain, epilepsy, Alzheimer's Disease, and Parkinson's Disease. This becomes even more important in America because at least 50% of the US population suffers from inadequate amounts of magnesium as a result of their diet—many without even knowing it. As smokers tend to be short in many nutrients dietarily, it is likely they need magnesium on a daily basis, even more so if you are American. For more information about magnesium, see Chapters 3, 4, 7-8, and 18.

EFAs

Essential Fatty Acids (EFAs) are included again in this section because fatty acids are critical to nerve health. First of all, every single cell in your body has a lipid bilayer protecting the cells while allowing cellular signaling in and out. Additionally, some nerves in your body are myelinated, which means there are deposits of fat located along the nerve itself. These fat deposits, or oligodendrocytes, increase the speed of nerve impulses. This is what allows folks to pull their hand back from the stove when it is hot. For more information on EFAs, see Chapters 4, 7, 9-10, 14, 17, and 19.

Botanicals

When looking at botanical medicine for this system, consider herbs that can act as nervines—herbs in support of the nervous system. This includes a number of herbs like Skullcap (Scutellaria), milky oats (*Avena sativa*), Catnip (Nepeta), Chamomile (*Matricaria chamomilla*), Valerian (Valeriana), and Hops (Humulus).

You may choose to support cognitive function with any of the following:

Ginkgo Biloba

Research has shown ginkgo can be safe and effective in regards to treating dementia. It seems to be most useful in cases of vascular dementia which is dementia due to problems with circulation and the small blood vessels of the brain. Additional studies have shown ginkgo can help with cognitive function and help balance out an anxious or depressed food. It has also been evaluated for supporting folks with Attention Deficit/Hyperactivity Disorder (ADHD), where it was found to be beneficial at a low dose. It's important to keep in mind most of these studies are small and more research needs to be done. Additional information about ginkgo biloba can be found in Chapter 10.

Gotu Kola

Gotu Kola (*Centella asiatica*) can also be used to support cognitive function. This is an adaptogenic herb meaning it can have a positive effect on many of the body's systems. Here, this potent herb is mentioned due to its action on the brain.

Ayurvedic medicine traditions use this herb to support the nerves and brain cells. Other Eastern modalities support that it is helpful for emotional concerns like depressed mood. It has also been shown to have anti-seizure properties as well, potentially reducing the number of seizures and decreasing their side effects. For more information about gotu kola, see Chapters 6 and 11.

Turmeric

Those who smoke should consider turmeric (*Curcuma longa*) because it is anti-inflammatory, antioxidant, antimicrobial, and has many anticancer mechanisms.

Oat

Overall, oat (*Avena sativa*) is great for many reasons, but it is included here because of its ability to help tonify the nervous system. Oats contain selenium which is an important cofactor for glutathione production to help deal with excessive oxidative damage caused by smoking. For more information about oat, see Chapters 10, 14, and 18.

Lifestyle

Diet

Refer to Chapters 3 and 4 for more detailed information on what a basic healthy diet entails and what it might look like for you. Additional things to keep in mind dietarily is to increase dark green leafy vegetables which are loaded with fiber and minerals. Beets can also be added in as they are very supportive of the cardiovascular system and smaller blood vessels present in the brain and other organs.

Other foods to consider are those which are rich in amino acids. Remember these are the basic building blocks of proteins in the body. The brain is no exception. It is dependent on amino acids to make hormones and neurotransmitters which allow our mind to communicate within our body. Essential fatty acids and the foods which are rich in them are also important to nerve health. This can be added in by consuming chia seeds, fish, nuts, etc.

Exercise

The concept of any movement is better than no movement returns here. The most important aspect of exercise for anyone to keep in mind is it should be something you like to do, and it should be something a little different or more than what you have been doing. Please refer to Chapters 7, 11, 12, 13, and 14 for more information on exercise, its many benefits, and how to incorporate it into your daily or weekly routine.

Other Therapies to Consider

There are many therapies supportive of nerve health including hydrotherapy which can be very useful for supporting the nervous system. More information about hydrotherapy can be found in Chapter 4 and complete instructions for several therapies are listed in the Apothecary chapter. Other therapies which may be helpful are listed below.

Meditation

Meditation is relatively commonplace today. When you think of meditation, you may think of a monk in a temple somewhere with legs crossed, eyes closed, and humming. This practice is much more than that, and there are many different ways to do it.

Science supports the benefit of meditation. A study compared a control group that did relaxation time versus an experimental group that participated in integrative mind-body exercises instead. Both groups showed improvements in autonomic nervous system function though results were much better in the experimental group. This benefit is supported by brain imaging. Meditation can be helpful with managing anxiety and stress, depression, and even addiction problems due to its implementation of brain imagery. It can also be helpful with pain management.

The practice of meditation can be as simple as sitting quietly and trying to keep your mind relaxed and clear of thoughts, repeating a mantra over and over, sitting in nature and just taking deep breaths, etc. There are apps you can download on your phone as a guide, and there are also videos you can check out online to learn more about meditation and what type of meditation practice may work for you.

Yoga

This practice was developed in India over 5,000 years ago. It was developed as a philosophical system to help people reach personal enlightenment, but nowadays it is a common exercise and mindful practice. Yoga has six different branches, each of which has a different philosophy and reasoning behind it. For example, Bikram yoga is also known as hot yoga, and there is Iyengar yoga which focuses on posture, etc.

Yoga can involve movement, breathing practices, or both, and it can help build strength, flexibility, and durability in the body. Different poses help focus the energy in your body in different ways to support overall health and well-being. It has been shown to be helpful and supportive in a wide variety of mental health concerns.

Forest Bathing

Shinrin-yoku or forest bathing is a practice formally coined as a term in Japan in the early 1980s. It has been shown to decrease blood pressure, overall stress, and it can even improve your immune system function. The practice itself is very simple and just involves going out for a walk in a nearby forested space. If you don't live near a forest, just spending time outside and away from the hustle and bustle of urban life can be helpful. The greener your space the better, as spending time with plants has been linked to a more positive mood.

Chapter 16:
What About The Gut?

Much of the gut is made up of little bacteria and other organisms that live and work communally. They produce nutrients for each other, consume one another's waste, and as a side-effect of these bacteria and other organisms living their lives, humans receive a functioning gut. This community is our microbiome and not only can it be damaged, but it can also stop working altogether. It is also possible to care for your gut, much as you would care for a pet! Feed it, clean it, care for it and it will love you unconditionally in return!

The gastrointestinal system is described in detail below, but basically, there is a tube that runs from your mouth to your anus and among the many things it does, its primary purposes are to help you get what you need to live (nutrients) and get rid of waste products. This part of the body is so important that holistic doctors consider it a cornerstone of health. If your gut is not healthy, you are not healthy.

The Gastrointestinal System

The gastrointestinal system is so critical to life, it begins forming in utero at three to four weeks of development; oftentimes this occurs before a woman even knows she's pregnant. The gastrointestinal system is how humans get nutrients from sources outside the body in order to fuel the cells and chemical reactions of life. This system starts at the mouth and tracks through the abdominal region all the way to the anus. It is made up of the mouth, pharynx (throat), esophagus, stomach, small intestine, large intestine, rectum, and anus.

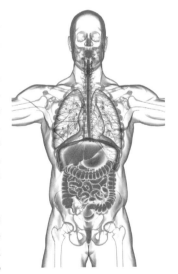

When you see food, your brain triggers enzyme and stomach acid production to begin in anticipation of digestion. Digestion is the process of breaking down food into much smaller parts to be absorbed and utilized in the body. It's important to realize food takes roughly 24 to 72 hours to be digested and eliminated from the system, and 10% of the calories you consume are used to fuel the process of digestion.

The first step of digestion is the mouth where food is chewed up, creating more surface area that makes food easier for our stomachs to break down. The food is also coated with saliva which contains some digestive enzymes that begin to break down the carbohydrates. Each swallow creates a bolus of food which is taken and moved through the esophagus by muscles that aren't under conscious control. The bolus travels down through the lower esophageal sphincter, the gateway to our stomach.

The stomach is a very acidic environment that breaks down proteins and kills any microbes ingested with the food. The food remains in the stomach for roughly a few hours as it is broken down into chyme, a liquid full of nutrients. This is slowly squirted into the duodenum, the first part of the human small intestine where the acidic chyme is mixed with bicarbonate to make it less acidic and no longer harmful to our intestines. Digestive enzymes to help further break down carbohydrates, fats, and proteins are also added here.

The nutrient-rich chyme slowly travels through the jejunum and ileum, the next two parts of the small intestine; from the stomach to the end of the small intestine generally takes 4-6 hours. The small intestine is where a significant portion of nutrients are absorbed, then the chyme travels through the ileocecal valve which divides the large intestine and small intestine. The large intestine continues some nutrient absorption, but it also absorbs water, concentrating the food into brown stools. These stools are then excreted through the anus when appropriate. The anus contains two sphincters, one which cannot be controlled and one which can, making it possible for humans to choose when they have bowel movements.

Additional organs which should be mentioned here include the liver, the gallbladder, and the pancreas. The liver makes bile salts which help break down fats and some vitamins. Bile salts are stored in the gallbladder which is a small pear-shaped organ nestled underneath the liver. The gallbladder contracts with fatty meals, squeezing bile into the small intestine when needed. The pancreas also makes enzymes to help break down carbohydrates, proteins, and fats. These enzymes are released into the small intestine via ducts. Please refer to Chapter 8 if you'd like to revisit information about the liver.

This entire process happens without much involvement on our part. Peristalsis, the organized constriction and contraction of muscles in our gastrointestinal tract, moves food and nutrients through the system at a steady pace.

How Smoking Damages the Gastrointestinal System

Now that you have a basic idea of how the gastrointestinal system works, let's dive into some specific damage that can occur due to smoking. Worldwide, it is estimated 5-10% of the human population has Irritable Bowel Syndrome (IBS). The risk of IBS goes up in all smokers, but the risk is highest in female smokers. This syndrome includes symptoms like cramping, abdominal pain, bloating, and gas. Stools are generally diarrhea or constipation or, in some cases, both. Additionally, smoking increases the risk of developing other intestinal disorders such as Crohn's disease or ulcers. New research has found smoking may also have a negative impact on the gut microbiome which may be why the risk of developing so many intestinal diseases goes up with smoking.

Smoking also increases the risk of developing an incisional hernia post-surgery by four times. This means that if you need to have abdominal surgery for any reason and you are a smoker, your risk of having surgical complications increases. In general, smoking significantly raises the risk of having surgical complications with any procedure. This includes the risk of infection, slow-healing wounds, etc., due, in part, to lower collagen synthesis. This means you can go in for routine surgery and leave with the risk of being worse off than you were when you went in.

Something else to consider, smoking can increase heartburn, one of the most common gastrointestinal complaints doctors see. Roughly 30% of all gastrointestinal symptoms reported in one survey were acid/heartburn related. It has been known for decades that nicotine can relax the lower esophageal sphincter, meaning it won't lock down as tight during digestion. This makes it easier for some of the acid in the stomach to leak, splashing back up into the esophagus to cause burning, upset stomach, and burping. Over time this can damage the throat and mouth depending on how severe the heartburn is.

How to Support and Heal the Gastrointestinal System

For smokers and non-smokers alike, the gut is often at the root of many health issues. Antibiotics, poor diets, illness, and stress are just a few things that can damage the GI tract. When you add smoking on top of normal, everyday life things, the gut becomes a major area of health focus.

Again, this is another great time to review Chapters 2-4, as they contain the basics of health that are referred to throughout this book and may help with your understanding of the information below. The items include general health information strategies that are incredibly useful for improving gut health.

Supplements

Psyllium Husk

Psyllium husk (*Plantago ovata*) is mentioned here because of the role fiber plays in overall gastrointestinal health. Fiber in general helps give feces form and allows the muscles in your intestinal tract to more easily move stool. It also binds with toxins and other substances such as cholesterol to carry them out of the body. This supports general detoxification and a healthy heart. Psyllium helps stools move more easily through the intestines by easing constipation and supporting a healthy gut microbiome. For more information about fiber, see Chapters 3, 8, 12, and 13.

Glutamine

Glutamine, also known as L-glutamine, is one of the most prevalent amino acids in the human body, and it just so happens it is also the primary fuel source of intestinal cells. This amino acid is generally regarded as conditionally essential because our glutamine needs can increase in times of trauma or disease. Glutamine helps promote the creation of more intestinal cells and helps prevent leaky gut by supporting strong and tight junction proteins. These junctions are the structures bonding intestinal cells together to keep germs, toxins, and other outside substances out of our bloodstream. Glutamine also helps keep inflammation down and protects cells from stresses which can lead to cellular death.

Research has shown glutamine can be helpful in reducing symptoms of some intestinal diseases such as Crohn's and IBS. If you decide to give it a try, powdered form is best. Typically it is recommended to start with 2-4 grams of powder mixed in water or juice 2-3 times a day between meals.

Digestive Enzymes

As mentioned in the description of the gastrointestinal system, the body makes stomach acid and digestive enzymes to help break down our food and allows for easier absorption. In cases of nutrient deficiencies or lowered "digestive fire", it can be helpful to supplement additional enzymes. Sometimes, the body is not able to adequately digest our food; humans need certain minerals and vitamins to produce enzymes and, for whatever reason, there may not be enough. This means your gastrointestinal system needs a little bit of support to help break down foods to get nutrients from them.

Digestive enzymes are one way this can be done. If you prefer boosting digestive enzyme production with food, try adding a teaspoon of apple cider vinegar or other vinegar to a couple of ounces of water and drinking it 10-15 minutes before a meal. If you do this, be sure to rinse your mouth out afterward, as the acid can harm tooth enamel over time. Otherwise, you can get digestive enzymes at any health food store. Follow the directions on the supplement bottle. Do not use a supplement that also includes HCl (hydrochloric acid a.k.a. stomach acid), unless you are doing so under your doctor's supervision. This is a potent substance and too much of it can damage the lining of the GI tract. There is no standard dosing because it varies greatly from one person to the next.

Botanicals

Ginger

Ginger is the rhizome of the plant *Zingiber officinale* which is known for supporting the gastrointestinal system. This is another herb used for thousands of years in Asia, especially in China. Traditionally, it has been used to treat colds, sore throats, fevers, infections, muscle aches and sprains, pain, migraines, etc. To support the gastrointestinal system, healers have used it for constipation, diarrhea, heartburn, burping, bloating, nausea, and vomiting among others. Ginger is anti-inflammatory, antioxidant, and can also help with ulcers.

Research strongly supports ginger as helpful with nausea and vomiting, especially in pregnant women. It can also help with nausea related to cancer treatments, surgery, or even exercise. It may also be helpful with fatty liver, inflammation in the gastrointestinal system, and with swallowing difficulties though more research is needed. This herb can be taken as a tea, lozenge or candy, capsules, or tincture. It can also be purchased from the grocery store and added fresh to recipes. This herb is very safe, even at higher doses, and doesn't have any known side effects or drug interactions.

Dandelion

Dandelion (*Taraxacum officinale*) is a herb long known in folklore medicine and is gaining strides in being understood by modern science. This herb is often most well known for its action on the liver, aiding the body in detoxification. It is also shown to have a healing and supporting action on the GI system. The leaf (diuretic, mildly stimulating to the liver) and root (bitter for the digestive system, liver tonic, detoxification support) are used in this plant. It can be enjoyed fresh in a garden salad, as a tea, tincture, or extract.

Peppermint

Peppermint (*Mentha piperita*) is a strong aromatic plant that grows in Europe, Asia, and North America. It aggressively spreads, so it's best grown in raised beds or containers to keep it under control. Peppermint has a sweetish smell and a warm pungent taste with a cool aftertaste. It can be used in cooking as an herb, and it is also used to flavor candy, desserts, and other culinary dishes. It is an antispasmodic herb which means it can help with stomach cramps, abdominal pain due to cramping, bloating, and farting. Research shows this can help relieve symptoms caused by IBS.

It can be helpful with tonifying and soothing the gastrointestinal tract, but it can cause heartburn as it relaxes the lower esophageal sphincter. If you suffer from heartburn regularly you should avoid using this herb unless you are under the care of a trained holistic health practitioner.

Calendula

Calendula (*Calendula officinalis*) is antioxidant, antimicrobial, and supports wound healing. Internally it can help move the lymph system, support fevers, and reduce muscle spasms—especially in the gastrointestinal tract. It is also very healing to superficial tissues, including the intestinal lining which is damaged in many intestinal diseases. For more information about calendula, see Chapters 6 and 11.

Lifestyle

Diet

What you put in your mouth is vitally important with any body system, but especially the gastrointestinal system. Leafy greens and colorful fruits in your diet provide a lot of trace nutrients and fiber. Many people get stuck in a rut eating the same few foods day in and day out which sets them up for a lack of nutrients. Each fruit and vegetable of a different color represents a different vitamin profile. Spices also play a role in nutrition. Herbs such as ginger and fennel are very supportive of your gastrointestinal health. Other spices include turmeric which is very anti-inflammatory and can help heal damaged tissues and oregano which is a great microbial to support a healthy microbiome. While the diet is discussed in numerous chapters of this book, an in-depth discussion can be found in Chapters 3 and 4.

- Fiber

  Fiber is probably one of the most important, if not the most critical part of food consumption to support a healthy gastrointestinal tract. For every 7 grams of fiber consumption, there is a significant reduction in the risk of developing cardiovascular disease. It is established that adequate fiber helps with IBS, IBD, diverticular disease, constipation, and more. The preferred method to get fiber is to consume whole foods with minimal processing. Adults should be getting at least 25 grams a day with 30 grams of fiber being the best, statistically, at supporting a healthy heart. If you can't get enough fiber through your diet, a supplement may help. For more information about fiber, see Chapters 3, 8, 12, and 13.

- Fermented Foods

  Fermented foods are also an important part of the dietary picture. Since humans first discovered fermentation, we've been eating these foods as a species. Fermented foods provide a more natural way for getting probiotics into the diet without taking yet another pill. If you prefer a food route to support your gut microbiome, it is recommended you try and incorporate more fermented foods in your diet such as kimchi, sauerkraut, water kefir, pickled vegetables (carrots, beets, cucumbers, etc.), kombucha, yogurt, milk, or kefir if dairy is tolerated, etc. Otherwise, you can buy probiotics at a health food store and most grocery stores. Remember, if you are immune compromised, you should avoid probiotics without a doctor's guidance and support. For more information about probiotics, see Chapters 4, 14-15, and 19.

- Food Sensitivities

  Eliminating food sensitivities is also helpful. This can be done by visiting your doctor for some testing, or you can do this at home. The simplest way at home is to do a dietary reset by eating just vegetables for 3 - 5 days, then going back through and adding in foods slowly. Add foods one at a time in a few servings one day, then watch for symptoms over the next two days—you'll be able to isolate a reaction if you have one. Food sensitivities can appear as low energy, headache, diarrhea, general malaise, etc. Your body is unique, and it is speaking to you subtly all the time if you are open to listening. Start with the most common foods that are linked to food sensitivities such as dairy, gluten, tree nuts, peanuts, and eggs.

Exercise

Exercise is always good to add in throughout your day. Movement tones muscles in your whole body including your abdomen which helps encourage healthy bowel movements. The tension in your abdominal muscles helps create pressure to keep stool moving through your system. Core training exercises and deep breathing exercises especially can help tone the stomach. Exercise doesn't have to be complex; walking and stretching are invaluable to getting your body moving and the blood flowing. Please refer to Chapters 7, 11, 12, 13, and 14 for more information on exercise, its many benefits, and how to incorporate it into your daily or weekly routine.

Other Therapies to Consider

Fasting

Fasting can be a powerful tool to help your body balance itself. It can help balance out blood sugars, lower inflammation, support heart and nervous system health, aid in weight loss, and even help optimize a healthy hormone balance. Fasting can be for a set number of hours, or it can be for several days depending on your health and health goals. One way you may be able to add fasting to your routine is through intermittent fasting. This means you refrain from eating for a certain number of hours during the day. Some people will just eat every day during a set time frame, such as 10 AM to 6 PM, or they may not eat for a whole day once a week. Fasting can be very dangerous if done improperly. Please seek assistance from your health practitioner if you are interested in fasting as it is not recommended for children, women during pregnancy, or those who are at risk of developing an eating disorder.

Constitutional Hydrotherapy

Constitutional hydrotherapy increases circulation throughout the body, and because of where the electrodes are located, it helps drive a deeper effect into the abdominal region. You can do this at home using hot and cold towels, and it is also effective at balancing out the gastrointestinal system. It supports the parasympathetic system to help boost digestion and relaxation. You can find instructions on a home version of this therapy in the Apothecary section or find a practitioner that offers this in their office. Read more about hydrotherapy in Chapter 4.

Massage, General and Abdominal

Massage therapy in general can be very helpful in supporting a healthy gastrointestinal tract. As it promotes relaxation, it supports regular bowel habits on a daily basis, and the more relaxed you are, the better your body can break down and absorb your foods.

Abdominal massage can be helpful for constipation, bloating, or gas in children and adults alike. It's important to do abdominal massage the right way; if you go the wrong direction, you can encourage stool to stay inside rather than moving down the tract for elimination. If this is done in the evening before bed, it encourages a morning bowel movement. For more information about abdominal massage see the Apothecary chapter.

Castor Oil Packs

Castor oil is very anti-inflammatory, and the warm heat of the pack helps drive this effect into your tissues. For your abdomen, this can be very relaxing and helpful for mild pain and discomfort. Plan on doing this for 30 - 60 minutes for the greatest effect. Refer to the Apothecary section or Chapters 3, 8, and 9 for more information.

Chapter 17:
Bones and Muscles

There is a great song called *Dry Bones* by The Delta Rhythm Boys. Part of the song goes like this:

Well, your toe bone connected to your foot bone

Your foot bone connected to your heel bone

Your heel bone connected to your ankle bone

Your ankle bone connected to your leg bone

Your leg bone connected to your knee bone

Your knee bone connected to your thigh bone

Your thigh bone connected to your hip bone

Your hip bone connected to your back bone

Your back bone connected to your shoulder bone

Your shoulder bone connected to your neck bone

Your neck bone connected to your head bone…

Remember, humans are built to move and are put together in a way that makes this task possible. The healthier the bones and muscles, the better we are able to move. The more we move, the healthier we are.

Bones form the skeleton and are held together by ligaments. Tendons connect the muscles to the bones. In the end, everything comes together to form a frame that holds the internal organs, and it is all covered by skin. Blood vessels and nerves run through every part of the body, including the bones and muscles which is a good thing! Bones and muscles are living and reshaping themselves as needed by the way we use them and care for them, or not. When we are doing something every day that introduces poison into the system, the muscles and bones are affected just like every other part of the body.

The Musculoskeletal System

The musculoskeletal system is composed of bones connected to each other with ligaments. Ligaments are very tough fibrous connective tissue. The human body contains 206 bones which give the body its shape. Bones also give the body protection such as the skull which wraps around the brain, or the ribs which shield the heart and lungs. Skeletal muscles are usually what someone thinks about when the word muscle is used. Humans have roughly 600 skeletal muscles in the body all working together. These are the muscles just under the skin which connect to the bones and allow for jumping, running, diving, crouching, walking, etc., throughout the day. Skeletal muscles are connected to the bones via tough connective tissue called tendons.

Muscles work like pulleys, shortening in length so the tendon can pull on the attached bone. The shortening is called contraction, and when the muscle is done firing, it relaxes and returns to its longer length. The nervous system signals muscles to contract and also helps coordinate movements into a cohesive flow so the actions are smooth and not jerky. The brain, spinal cord, and nerves send signals to and from the muscles, and the more you move/exercise, the more coordinated muscle contractions become. When this system is functioning as it should, we can move pain-free, with ease

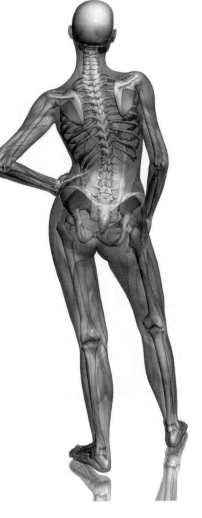

for relatively long distances. We are also able to lift and push, pull and twist, jump and run, again with little pain. There may be discomfort after such exercise, as in sore or tired muscles, but the body recovers.

When something has gone wrong, there are symptoms. The muscles hurt or ache and exhaust quickly with little effort. Joints can be painful and noisy and may become red or inflamed. Chronic hip, back, knee, or neck complaints may pop up and persist regardless of various treatments. Running, jumping, climbing, pushing, pulling, all of these become a dreaded activity. For smokers, there are a few particular dangers to try and support the body through when it comes to the musculoskeletal system.

How Smoking Damages the Musculoskeletal System

Smoking has been found to have negative impacts on the musculoskeletal system, especially the bones. It doesn't matter whether you are younger or older, male or female, the bones will suffer in smokers. Bone mass density was found to be lower in almost every study evaluating this information, increasing the risk of fracture. One study, looking at adolescent females, concluded that starting smoking at age 13 affected bone growth, and it was associated with a lower average bone mass density at age 17. Other studies supported this conclusion.

Postmenopausal women who smoked were found to have significantly lower bone density than those who did not smoke and were at an increased risk for falling. Smoking is also hard on the teeth. In smokers, there is increased periodontal disease, bone loss, and missing teeth when compared to non-smokers. Men are also at increased risk of low bone density, especially those who also suffer from Chronic Obstructive Pulmonary Disease (COPD). In those with COPD, men had up to 84% greater risk of having low bone density in their spine. Men also tend to have more vertebral fractures than women with low bone density. This is multifactorial, but smokers have higher oxidants, lower antioxidants, lower parathyroid hormone (bone-building hormone), vitamin D, a higher calcium excretion, and a lower concentration of bone marrow progenitor cells, and proteins which are needed to build bones.

There are a many things to be found in the research:

- Rheumatoid arthritis (RA), an autoimmune disease, in smokers was found to have a higher rate of disability with more severe joint changes; smokers also took more drugs to help manage the disease
- Smokers with osteoarthritis were also found to have higher reported pain scores
- With regard to muscles, smokers were found to have more oxidative fiber atrophy, meaning their muscles were not as strong as compared to non-smokers
- Surgeries to repair or replace joints had a higher risk of complications after the surgery

Additionally, the impact smoking has on the cardiovascular system can make matters worse. Muscles depend on the blood to get oxygen, and not only does smoking interfere with oxygen delivery levels (refer to Chapters

6 and 7 for more information), it impairs the body's ability to maintain your capillaries. Capillaries are small blood vessels that deliver oxygen and nutrients directly to the muscles, and smoking reduces the number of capillaries in the body over time.

How to Support and Heal the Musculoskeletal System

Both the muscles and bones need blood and the nutrients it carries to function. Muscles and bones also need to get rid of toxins and metabolic by-products (the normal everyday toxicity produced simply by living), just like the rest of the body. In other words, they need to detoxify, and blood and lymph play a huge role here just as they do with the rest of the body. While the muscles and bones share these needs, they have some special needs of their own.

Bone requires a full spectrum of nutrients like protein, fats, and carbohydrates, but it also needs all the macro- and micronutrients, vitamins, minerals, and water. Bones thrive, are dense, strong, and replenish themselves regularly, especially with nutrients such as Vitamin D, Calcium, Protein, Magnesium, Vitamin B, Vitamin K, Vitamin A, and Zinc.

It is interesting to point out that many people with healthy bones do not necessarily take these nutrients as supplements, nor do they weigh their diet heavily in foods providing these nutrients. So, what is going on? Research shows that the nutritional status of the body is important for the bones, but it is more than nutrients that are critical to bone health. Proper posture is very important, so there is good nervous system interaction and sufficient blood circulation. This feeds the bones and moves waste away. Humans need to be active—movement is key and the musculoskeletal system must be used every day. Humans have to move, and the more they move, although not to excess, the healthier the bones (and muscles). When we exercise, the attachment between muscle and bone is strengthened, the body sends nutrients and fluids to where the body needs them, and the system is energized. A relatively healthy diet and proper elimination are present in people with good bone health.

Muscles also have their own special nutrient needs, such as glutamine. This is an amino acid that helps repair muscle, support gut health, and is important for immune health. Protein in the diet is essential as it provides this and other amino acids needed by your muscles. Another nutrient important to muscles is vitamin C as it is essential for connective tissue repair throughout the entire body.

Here you can see that the health of your body can be elevated as a whole by doing the basics. The following information may be quite different from what you would typically think. Instead of thinking every smoker should be taking calcium, focus on your bones and muscles and how you can support them overall so you have a good strong frame.

Supplements

The musculoskeletal system relies on a lot of the same basic nutrients as other systems. A good quality multivitamin and mineral formula helps make sure there are adequate B vitamins. B12 and folate are critical as they are cofactors needed by muscle cells to make repairs. For more information about B vitamins, see Chapters 4, 8, 11-12, 14, and 18.

Trace Minerals

Many trace minerals can be helpful for bone health. Boron is needed for bone development and regeneration. It positively impacts Vitamin D usage in the body, and it helps lower the excretion of calcium and magnesium in postmenopausal women. This means those minerals are being absorbed and used by the body rather than passing right through. Copper, manganese, and zinc are also important for bone health. Animal models with deficient amounts of trace minerals have shown thinner thigh bones than those given adequate nutrition. More information about minerals can be found in Chapters 3 and 4, and are discussed throughout most chapters of this book.

Essential Fatty Acids

Essential fatty acids (EFAs), in addition to having wide-ranging benefits on mental health and nervous system function, are also supportive of having healthy muscles. There are reports of older adults taking EFAs, specifically omega-3s, showing improved muscle strength and size. EFAs also appear to be protective of muscles in instances where they aren't being used as often such as recovery from an injury or in elders who have balance problems. For more information on EFAs, see Chapters 4, 7, 9-10, 14-15, and 19.

Bone Support

These are particular supplements filled with nutrients essential to bone health. Bone support supplements are great to add in, but if you are already taking a few supplements such as a multivitamin or trace mineral formula, you have to make sure you aren't getting too much of certain nutrients and not enough of others. For example, you may be taking a multivitamin, vitamin D, and a bone supplement. If all three of those contain Vitamin D, it's your job to add up all the IUs of vitamin D and make sure it's not too much. It is possible to overdose on vitamins, making it too much of a good thing. Specific nutrients to track are vitamin A, B vitamins, vitamin K, calcium, magnesium, and zinc. Don't forget to add in the nutrients which you are getting from your diet as well, because everything adds up.

Additionally, when you take several different supplements, there can be interference with absorption. An example of this is iron, copper, and zinc. They are all absorbed through the same receptor in the intestines, and if you are taking lots of zinc, you may not be absorbing enough copper or iron which leads to deficiency over time. Working with a nutritionist or doctor familiar with nutritional therapies can be helpful with this.

Protein

Protein is what muscles are made of, and having adequate amounts in your diet is essential. In the case of athletes or elders who don't eat a lot of food, adding a protein supplement can be helpful. There are many different protein sources out there, and I recommend using a simple protein blend with fewer additives. It should also be organic-based whenever possible. You can get animal-based protein powders like whey or egg, or you can get plant-based powders such as pea, hemp, soy, or brown rice. These powders can be added to a smoothie loaded with vegetables or dark berries for antioxidants, or they can be mixed with water. Remember, this is adjunctive and most of your protein should be coming out of your diet.

Botanicals

There are a number of nutritive herbs that you can include in your diet to help support bone and muscle health.

Red Clover

Red Clover (*Trifolium pratense*), discussed in Chapter 9, has been shown to be promising for the support of bone density. One year of daily supplementation decreased the loss of bone density in the lumbar (lower) spine of pre- and perimenopausal women. Another study tracked a group of menopausal women for twelve weeks who supplemented with red clover. Many displayed positive changes in their lumbar bone density.

Red clover can be taken as a tea, capsule, or tincture. Research studies find positive effects with concentrations of isoflavones at 30 mg or more per dose. As this is a slower-acting herb, you can take it once daily for at least three months though it is well-tolerated for longer-term use. This herb should not be used in pregnant women.

Alfalfa

Alfalfa (*Medicago sativa*) is another plant commonly used in farming similar to red clover. It contains high amounts of vitamins, minerals, and phytoestrogens. It's a good source of calcium, potassium, phosphorus, iron, and vitamins A, C, E, and K. It has been used for high cholesterol, diabetes, and indigestion. It can also affect other health conditions, but research is still ongoing.

Of particular interest to smokers, alfalfa has been shown to improve inflammation and oxidative damage caused by nicotine. Alfalfa can be added to soups and salads as it is easy to grow as sprouts in a window. It can also be taken as a capsule, tincture, or tea. As always, it is recommended to look for organic sources or even grow them yourself at home whenever possible.

Lifestyle

Diet

While the diet is discussed in numerous chapters of this book, an in-depth discussion can be found in Chapters 3 and 4. As always, a whole-foods-based diet low in processed foods is going to be your best bet for a healthy musculoskeletal system. This should include a variety of vegetables and fruits of all different colors. Including dark berries. One study found having a quarter cup of antioxidant-rich blackberries daily was helpful in reducing smoking-induced bone loss. High-quality proteins including grass-fed beef, fresh fish, free-range chicken, turkey, etc., will provide the basic building blocks your body needs to maintain its skeletal structure.

Most importantly, making sure you get calcium-rich foods is paramount to having healthy bones. It is possible to get all of your calcium from supplements, but research shows this drastically increases your risk of developing cardiovascular disease. Calcium supplementation shouldn't exceed 500 mg daily and the rest of your daily calcium intake (1,000 mg for the average adult) should come from whole food sources. These foods are great calcium sources: milk, milk alternatives, yogurt, cheese, cottage cheese, ricotta cheese, broccoli, kale, mustard greens, collard/turnip greens/spinach, tofu, beans, salmon, sardines, dry cereal, hot cereal, English muffin, almonds, sesame seeds, molasses, navy beans, and chickpeas.

Exercise

Exercise is very important to bone and muscle health. Anything you are physically capable of doing to get movement into your day counts as exercise and is better than what you may have been doing before. You can walk, swim, bike, do resistance training, etc. Specifically for bone health and osteoporosis concerns, adding weight-bearing exercise improves bone density more than non-weight-bearing exercise. This can be as simple as adding a full water bottle to a backpack and going for a walk around the block, especially if you don't enjoy going to the gym or lifting weights. If you are going to add in weights, then working with a trainer is highly recommended. They can teach you proper lifting techniques and give you a personalized workout regimen to incorporate into your routine. It's very easy to lift wrong or lift too much too early and having the help of a professional will go a long way! If you are not already exercising, be sure to check in with your doctor before beginning any new program. Please refer to Chapters 7, 11-14, and 16 for more information on exercise, its many benefits, and how to incorporate it into your daily or weekly routine.

Other Therapies to Consider

Detoxification

Consistent and gentle detoxification with good liver and kidney support is important for healthy bones. See Chapter 8 for a more detailed discussion of detoxification.

Chapter 18:
The Master Reset: Sleep

Sleep is essential for physical, mental, and emotional health. When asleep the body relaxes into a different state and many important things happen. For one, the body does most of its healing at this time. The neurotransmitters can settle down and the organ systems can reset. Sleep lightens the burden on the adrenal and thyroid glands, both of which are in a constant state of high demand during our waking hours. During sleep, the psyche can process the enormous amount of information taken in during the day. Without adequate sleep, you cannot be well.

In today's society, whether you are a smoker or not, adults and children alike are spending more time awake late at night to study, work, or have fun. All those late nights may be slowly killing us. More than twenty years of research reveals that sleep is vitally important to all aspects of health. When you add smoking into the mix, this creates a body full of substances to be detoxified and systems to be healed.

The amount of sleep needed varies based on an individual's general state of health, age, activity level, quality of sleep, and genetics (e.g., some people really are night owls). Infants typically require 14-15 hours of sleep per 24-hour period, young children about 12 hours, teens roughly 9 hours, and most adults need 7-9 hours. Here's a general rule of thumb for determining your sleep requirement: If you don't feel refreshed when you wake up, you probably aren't getting enough sleep.

So, the big question in your mind right now might be, how affected is a smoker when it comes to sleep? Turns out, it is pretty significant. The American Sleep Association (ASA) tells us:

> Smokers take longer to fall asleep and wake up more frequently, they sleep less than nonsmokers, and have a less deep sleep. Because of this, smokers are more likely to wake up feeling tired and not well rested. Smoking can cause insomnia, which is the inability to fall asleep or stay asleep.

So, how does a smoker support themselves to get their best sleep? Let's start with a brief and general overview of the human sleep system.

The Sleep System

Sleep is something every creature on the planet utilizes in some way, shape, or form. In humans, sleep is when the body rests and restores itself. There are two types of sleep including non-rapid eye movement (non-REM) and rapid eye movement (REM) sleep. Non-REM sleep happens first and includes three stages of sleep with the second and third stages being the most restful. It is during non-REM that your body is repairing itself. REM sleep occurs roughly 60 - 90 minutes after falling asleep, and this is when you tend to have dreams. The stages cycle in order from the first stage of non-REM sleep through REM sleep, then it starts at the first stage again. A full sleep cycle takes roughly 1.5 to 2 hours. The longer you are able to sleep, the more REM sleep you'll have, and less deep sleep. The older you get, the less and less non-REM and REM sleep you get, which is why adults do not sleep as deeply as children.

Most of what is known about sleep and health comes from studies of what happens to the mind and body when there hasn't been enough or any sleep. There are many ongoing studies, but here are some of the major findings to date in animal and human research:

- Living without sleep for even a few months results in death
- Sleeping fewer than eight hours a night on a regular basis is associated with increased risk for diabetes, heart disease and stroke, depression, colds and flu, and obesity
- Sleep affects brain chemistry and has an important role in the functioning of the nervous, immune, and endocrine systems
- During sleep, a person develops and reinforces neural pathways involved in memory, learning, and emotion
- New research suggests sleep helps flush toxins from the brain

While asleep, the body manufactures and releases hormones to repair damage caused by stress and the environment in which you live, work, and play. The hormones are then used by the body, night and day. For example, growth hormone, which is primarily released at night, is used to cleanse the liver, build muscle, break down fat, and normalize blood sugar. If a person isn't getting sufficient sleep, it is common for them to get sick more often and take longer to recover. Lack of sleep also increases inflammation which has been linked to heart disease and stroke.

Skimping on shut-eye is linked with obesity in adults and children. This is because a lack of sleep interferes with the levels of ghrelin and leptin, metabolic hormones that signal when you're hungry and when you're full. Lack of sleep also disrupts cortisol which, at proper levels, helps balance blood sugar.

You don't have to pull all-nighters to become sleep deprived. A sleep debt of just one to two hours a few nights a week can affect your health and performance. To become fully well-rested and regain energy after a sleep debt, get an extra hour of sleep each night for one week.

If you experience any of the following, you may be sleep deprived.

- Daytime drowsiness
- General fatigue
- Poor memory and difficulty concentrating
- Changes in appetite
- Difficulty dealing with stress
- Irritability
- Muscle tension
- Impaired vision
- Increase in accidents or clumsiness

How Smoking Damages the Sleep System

When you consider how smoking affects one's ability to get proper amounts and quality of sleep, you should consider both the direct and indirect effects. Here is an example of an indirect effect: Consider a family that does not earn enough money for the basics of life. Cigarettes are expensive. Often, there is a constant sense of guilt because they know their money could be used for their family. And to make matters worse, they not only use money they don't really have, but they are using it to create illness in their body which will cost them in the long run. Now, they might not think of this every waking moment; in fact, it is probably buried deep in their psyche. When asleep, these deep, suppressed ideas can surface and disturb their rest.

The direct effects of smoking on sleep include difficulty falling asleep and an increased risk of excessive daytime sleepiness, non-restorative sleep, and trouble getting up in the morning. Men in particular seem to be at a higher risk of having disturbing dreams which prevents them from getting quality sleep. Insomnia and sleep apnea tend to occur more often in smokers versus non-smokers as well. One theory about why smoking has such a negative effect on sleep is that smokers go into small withdrawals every night while they are sleeping; nicotine withdrawal in smokers trying to quit and former smokers consistently causes sleep disturbances.

This is a really important system, and it must be taken care of. Something all doctors know and rarely ever argue about is how important sleep is for human beings. Read on to take a look at ways you can support yourself and get better quality sleep.

How to Support and Heal the Sleep System

Keep in mind as long as you smoke, the following suggestions just help keep the hole in the dam plugged. Meaning, if you are smoking and stimulating your system with nicotine, then using a calming and relaxing herb to sleep, you are temporarily fixing what will be a more serious problem later. Focus instead on the core principles of health which include helping your body clear itself of toxins and taking in the nutritive substances you need to heal.

Consider revisiting Chapter 8 because other than quitting, supporting your body as it tries to heal from the damage of smoking may be one of the best ways to improve your sleep.

Supplements

Something I have found through the last 17 years in many of my patients is how a high state of oxidative stress seems to go hand in hand with sleeping troubles. My observations led me to believe that as their oxidized state lessens their sleep improves. In science that is called a correlation, and in clinical practice, reliable correlations guide practitioners on how to help others more quickly. The following supplements may be surprising. Examples include melatonin or 5-HTP which many natural medicine doctors almost always include in their treatment plans. But remember, the goal is not to treat insomnia, it is to restore the body to a better state of health given the influx of daily toxins from smoking. Again, the best thing to do is to support the overall health of the system and allow the body to heal itself.

Vitamin C

Vitamin C is a potent antioxidant that tends to be low in smokers. By adding this into your routine, you are supporting soft tissue production as well as a healthy sleep pattern. For more information about Vitamin C, see Chapters 3-4, 6-9, 11, and 19.

Magnesium

Magnesium is a critical mineral utilized in more than 300 chemical reactions in the body. It can also help relax tight muscles which may be contributing to poor sleep. One study looked at sleep quality in elderly individuals. Researchers in this study found increasing magnesium intake lowered cortisol (stress hormone) and increased melatonin. Patients in the study were also able to get to sleep faster and feel more rested when they awoke. For more information about magnesium, see Chapters 3, 4, 7-8, and 15.

Glutathione

Glutathione has been discussed several times as the master molecule of the oxidative state of humans, something consistently low in smokers. Researchers have found in people with insomnia or poor sleep, antioxidant molecules are lower, and in people with lower antioxidants sleep is poorer. Glutathione is included here because of the relationship between antioxidant status and quality of sleep, especially given smokers tend to run low on this substance. For more information on glutathione see Chapters 4, 6, 8, and 10.

B Vitamins

Remember B vitamins come as a complex. Vitamins B1 and B2 help the body produce melatonin, the sleep hormone. Vitamin B6 helps with your thinking ability, supports immune health, and helps your body produce serotonin for mood and melatonin for sleep support. B12 helps your body produce red blood cells, supports brain and cardiovascular functions, and appears to regulate your circadian rhythm (research is currently ongoing). Smokers tend to run low on B vitamins which can lead to sleep issues. If you decide to add this to your regimen, take B vitamins with breakfast or lunch at the very latest. They can be stimulating enough to cause sleep disturbances in some people if taken too late in the day. For more information about B vitamins, see Chapters 4, 8, 11-12, 14, and 17.

Botanicals

Liver Support

The liver has many functions in the body, including detoxification and hormone balancing. In regards to sleep, it helps make sure stress hormones are being adequately addressed and broken down as needed. To support this process, there are liver supplement options. You can read more about how to support your liver in Chapter 8.

Ashwagandha

Ashwagandha (*Withania somnifera*) has been shown to be a potent antioxidant. It is anti-inflammatory, neuroprotective, supportive of and expands memory capabilities, increases sleep health, can help with anxious mood, and is blood-supporting.

Research has shown ashwagandha can lower cortisol which has been shown to be higher in smokers, especially those smoking ten or more cigarettes daily. It also helps improve sleep quality, helps with anxiety, eating behaviors, and mental wellness in overweight or obese adults. Researchers have found at doses of 300 mg twice a day, it is well tolerated. It can improve sleep quality and sleep onset latency, especially in those with insomnia. There is also promising research on how it can potentially support people with anxiety and insomnia, though further investigation is needed.

Oat

Oat (*Avena sativa*) can be helpful due to its relaxing and calming properties. A bath or cup of milky oat seed tea in the evening can help with winding down and preparing your body for sleep. For more information about oat, see Chapters 10 and 14-15.

Lavender

Lavender (*Lavandula angustifolia*) is a richly scented, deep purple flower, native to the mountainous zones of the Mediterranean, but widely available throughout the U.S., Europe, and Australia. Over 2,500 years ago, the ancient Egyptians used lavender in rituals, including the mummification process. In ancient Greece and Rome, the flowers and oils were sold at premium prices for use in soaps, perfumes, and natural remedies.

Today, lavender essential oil is used in aromatherapy to help balance and soothe mental and emotional stress. While lavender initially feels reviving to the senses, within moments, it has a calming and restorative effect. In botanical medicine, lavender is used in treatment for anxiety, insomnia, fatigue, tension headache, and mild depression. For individuals with ADHD or Autism Spectrum Disorders, lavender is safe to use as part of a relaxation routine. It's one of the few essential oils that may be applied directly to the skin undiluted or in combination with other oils for massage and bathing.

Lavender is available as a tincture, infusion, extract, or as an essential oil used alone or in combination with other relaxing herbs. Dried lavender and its derivatives are used in bath salts, sachets, eye pillows, and potpourris. Lavender, in loose herb form, may also be used in herbal beverages and teas.

Lifestyle

Diet
It's important to eat a light last meal of the day. A small dinner eaten 2-3 hours before sleep is ideal. A full stomach interferes with sleep as the body works at digestion. If you need a bedtime snack, combine a carbohydrate and protein, such as almond butter on toast, Greek yogurt with sugar-free granola, or cheese and crackers. Avoid products containing caffeine, sugar, or nicotine as their effects can last several hours. While the diet is discussed in numerous chapters of this book, an in-depth discussion can be found in Chapters 3 and 4.

Exercise
Natural light helps regulate the hormones that promote ideal sleep-wake patterns. Open the curtains as early as possible and get outdoors during the day to increase light exposure. Also, exercising during the day or early evening makes it easier to fall asleep and increases the amount of deep sleep obtained. Please refer to Chapters 7, 11-14, and 16-17 for more information on exercise, its many benefits, and how to incorporate it into your daily or weekly routine.

Other Therapies to Consider

Hydrotherapy (Constitutional, Contrast, or Heating Compress)
If you cannot locate a local practitioner who does constitutional hydrotherapy, consider contrast or heating compress hydrotherapy done at home. You will get the most benefit from this therapy if you can incorporate it into a weekly practice. Hydrotherapy is discussed in more detail in Chapter 4 and you can find specific instructions on how to do it at home in the Apothecary Chapter.

Detoxification

Consistent and gentle detoxification with good liver and kidney support can help promote sleep. See Chapter 8 for a more detailed discussion of detoxification.

Sleep Meditation

Moving your meditation practice right before bed can help you relax your body and mind, calm your emotions, may help you fall asleep more quickly, and sleep more deeply. There are different kinds of sleep meditation such as guided or unguided, and with or without music. You can try out different ones until you find the best fit. For additional information on meditation please refer back to Chapter 15.

Tips For A Good Night's Sleep

These are not typically considered therapy, but they can be extremely helpful.

- *In the sack for sleep and sex only.* Regular sex can improve sleep quality so don't use your time between the sheets to deal with daily hassles—take that outside of the bedroom (or record it in a journal). If you don't feel sleepy, leave the room and do something relaxing until you feel drowsy. Then, go back to bed.

- *Set a sleep schedule.* This includes a soothing pre-sleep routine, such as a warm bath, reading, or gentle yoga. Go to bed and wake up at the same time each day. This entrains your body rhythms, making it easier to fall asleep. If you need a nap, get it in before 5:00 PM and limit yourself to 20 minutes.

- *Surround yourself with a cave-like ambiance.* A sleeping space should be quiet, dark, and cool (between 60-72 degrees Fahrenheit or 15.56-22.22 degrees Celsius). If you work at night, use blackout shades or an eye mask to reduce sunlight. Remove electronic devices, computers and TVs from your room, as research shows the use of digital devices within an hour before going to bed has a negative effect on sleep quality.

Chapter 19:
Your Defenses

You have arrived at the last system discussed in this book. Up to this point, the picture has been one of an interconnected body in which all parts must work together to create a healthy enough state. The immune system is no different. It is part of the body, it is all over the body, and when there are things that need to be healed, it participates as a key player. If your immune system is overactive and seems to be attacking your body, or it is underactive and not responding as it should, there is always a reason. Unless the body has all the nutrients it needs, is removing toxins, and healing is being supported, it is not healthy enough. When the body is not healthy enough, there are symptoms.

Because smoking introduces a constant source of toxins, the body needs to be supported in extra ways every day. Let's take a look at the immune system, what goes wrong in smokers, and learn some ideas of how to support the body.

The Immune System

The immune system a.k.a. 'The Great Defender' is uniquely designed to keep a human healthy and fend off illness and infection. It is made up of organs, including the skin, lungs, and gut, as well as specialized cells. The immune system's job is to remain on alert for disease-causing invaders and to protect the body against them.

The human immune system's first responders are white blood cells (WBC) that are alerted to the presence of an invader. Some WBCs seek and destroy invaders while others have a cellular memory that enables the body to remember and recognize previous invaders. This allows known invading cells and viruses to be recognized and destroyed faster when they are reintroduced to the body. For example, if you get chickenpox, your body develops immunity to the virus; if you're exposed to chickenpox again, you won't contract it.

Sometimes cellular communication goes haywire, and the immune system starts attacking healthy cells in the body. This is called an autoimmune response; it can lead to autoimmune disease of which there are many types including Hashimoto's Thyroiditis or Rheumatoid Arthritis. There are also conditions, such as Selective IgA Deficiency, where some part of the immune response is lacking or not functioning properly.

Each person's immune system is as unique as their individual family health history, lifestyle, and environmental conditions. Some folks seem to never get sick, while others catch every bug going around. The strength of the immune system also changes as you age. Because the immune system is the greatest defender against disease, it's critical to keep it strong, healthy, and balanced.

This is a complex system with many parts all interconnected with other systems throughout the body, in addition to the direct toxic effects on the cells and organs of the immune system. The most significant work done in understanding the effect of smoking on the immune system comes from the field of psychoneuroimmunology where the intricate connection between the psyche, nervous, and immune system is explored.

How Smoking Damages the Immune System

The toxins introduced into the body when smoking directly damages the immune system including decreased levels of cells such as;

- Natural killer cells (NK cells), special cells that help clear cancer from the body
- Immunoglobulins, cells important in a variety of immune system function
- T helper cells (Th1/Th2/Th17), CD4+CD25+ regulatory T cells, CD8+ T cells, B cells and memory T/B lymphocytes
- Macrophages, cells that help clean up the immune system debris

Researchers have been able to show, in addition to directly decreasing immune function, smoking causes changes in the body that increase the risk for cancer—this makes sense since proper immune function is required to keep the body clear of cancer cells. There can also be increased inflammation lingering throughout the body because the cells of the immune system help clear inflammatory byproducts. The immune system also relies on properly functioning systems such as the ones already discussed including the respiratory, cardiovascular, detoxification, and nervous system. As the other systems function better, so does the immune system.

How to Support and Heal the Immune System

The first step in supporting immunity lies in creating a general state of wellness. The body was built so perfectly that the really important processes, like the immune system, will start running better and be more functional with even just a little bit of fine-tuning—as long as it is the correct fine-tuning. One error often made in the field of medicine is to ask a part of the body to do something it can no longer do well because the other systems it relies on are not functioning. So while there are suggestions in this section to support your immune system, consider that it would all work so much better with an improvement in lifestyle choices. As you know by now, when you smoke, you introduce toxins that affect your entire body. If you smoke daily, you have to work on your basic health every day.

Supplements

Probiotics

These are used to help maintain a healthier gut and therefore a healthier immune system. Remember, 80% of your immune system is located in your gut, so having balanced intestinal flora is a major factor in defending your body against disease. Balanced gastrointestinal (GI) flora is critical to the functioning of the immune system, synthesis of nutrients, and detoxification. Smoking can directly disturb the gut flora and as a result, a constant supply of healthy and thriving organisms is needed for your gut to thrive. For more information about probiotics, see Chapters 4 and 15-16.

Minerals

Minerals are needed for every reaction in the body including building and maintaining a healthy and properly functioning immune system. Whether to boost or lessen its function, without having a full complement and steady supply of minerals, the immune system will falter. Smoking depletes minerals from the body, and therefore, they need to be regularly replaced. Magnesium is critical to maintaining your healthy enough self. More information about minerals can be found in Chapters 3 and 4 as well as discussed throughout most chapters of this book.

Essential Fatty Acids (EFAs)

EFAs are also depleted when smoking. Studies in which EFAs were supplemented in smokers showed a drop in oxidative stress. This makes sense because EFAs are critical for properly functioning nervous and immune systems. For more information on EFAs, see Chapters 4, 7, 9-10, 14-15, and 17.

Vitamin C

Smokers consistently have lower levels of Vitamin C as compared to non-smokers. Those who smoke are at even greater risk for developing severe deficiency if they are not adequately supplementing. Vitamin C is incredibly important for immune function. Typically, those who smoke should start to take 500 mg of Vitamin C several times a day. This can be done through food, chewable tablets, capsules, or drinks. Almost every single person, after taking Vitamin C for a few days, feels a difference. The body is better able to deal with oxidative stress and can start doing some tissue repair. Eating fresh, uncooked, and unprocessed foods high in C is a great way to keep your levels up. Alternatively, there are many products on the market such as chewables, capsules, and liquids to help you get enough of this vitamin. For more information about Vitamin C, see Chapters 3-4, 6-9, 11, and 18.

Botanicals

In addition to the following herbs, the recipe for Immune Tea is included in the Apothecary section. This is a tasty blend of several herbs including lemon balm, oat straw, elderberry, hibiscus, rose hips, astragalus, and ginger. Ideally, you would drink one to two cups of tea daily starting in early fall and throughout the winter. For those with a struggling immune system, this tea should be drunk year-round.

Osha

Osha (*Ligusticum porteri*) grows in the Rocky Mountains and parts of Mexico. It has been traditionally used by Hispanic and Native American peoples to support the immune system, stimulate appetite, and help with gastrointestinal complaints like indigestion and vomiting. It has been used to support the body with colds and flus, sore throats, and fevers.

One of the effects of smoking is a direct increase of oxidative damage in the body. Osha has been shown to not only increase the substances in the body needed to clear this kind of damage but to also directly reduce the damaging factors. In herbal medicine the root is used, typically in a tincture form, and a standard dose is 1-5 ml, 2-3 times a day.

Elderberry

Elderberry (*Sambucus nigra*) prefers growing in moist, shady areas in Europe, Asia, and North Africa. It's also been naturalized in North America.

It is most often found growing as part of the underbrush in forests. Various parts of the plant were traditionally used with the berries being most prominent in modern times. Elderberry has been commonly used as a food, wine, or pie, and has also been used as a flavoring or dye.

Elderberry has been looked at extensively for its usefulness in supporting immune function in the human body. While there are some conflicting findings in certain populations; in general, this herb can help support and not overstimulate the immune system. Elderberries are rich in vitamin C and flavonoids that act as antioxidants and exhibit anti-inflammatory properties. Studies have shown that elder extracts may inhibit the replication of viruses. The berries are used for medicine and if harvested fresh, must be dried before making them into teas, extracts, or tinctures. There are a number of products available, but one of the best ways to add this to your daily life is as a tea.

Garlic

Garlic (*Allium sativa*) also acts in an immune-supportive manner. Known widely as the "stinking rose," garlic is a member of the lily family. It is cultivated worldwide and is a key ingredient in global cuisine including Chinese, French, Thai, Cajun, and Italian cooking. The use of garlic as food and medicine has been documented for thousands of years. Its medicinal effectiveness and versatility have stood the test of time and garlic remains widely used in Chinese, Ayurvedic, and Naturopathic medical practices.

Garlic is a nutritional powerhouse, with a wide range of trace minerals including selenium, chromium, potassium, germanium, calcium, and iron, as well as vitamins A, C, and B complex. In addition to providing an assortment of micronutrients, garlic has a multitude of phytonutrients with active medicinal properties including at least 23 sulfur compounds, the most active of which is allicin. Allicin and other sulfur compounds produced in its breakdown have extensive antimicrobial activity, inhibiting the growth of many bacterial and fungal organisms.

Along with its antimicrobial properties, garlic also has numerous protective effects for the cardiovascular system. Studies show that regular consumption of 1-2 cloves of garlic per day can improve cholesterol and triglyceride levels. In addition, garlic supplements have proven useful for decreasing plaque formation in blood vessel walls. Garlic is also used to reduce blood pressure, decrease the likelihood of blood clots, and modestly reduce blood glucose levels.

Some chemical constituents of garlic have also been examined for their ability to inhibit certain cancer-causing nitroso compounds. Consuming both raw and cooked garlic has been correlated with lower rates of stomach, intestinal, and other cancer types. It can be incorporated easily through your diet otherwise, supplements are widely available.

Lifestyle

Diet

As mentioned time and again, it's important to review the healthy diet basics found in Chapters 3 and 4. Focus on minimizing caffeine and sugar which is proinflammatory and suppressive to the immune system. You should also try to eliminate food additives, colorings, fried foods, items identified as a food allergen or sensitivity, and over-processed or GMO foods. All of these have been linked in some way to less than optimal immune function.

Fermented foods can help support gut health which is important for proper immune function. Research shows fermented foods positively affect the gut microbiome by supporting beneficial bacteria which can improve immune health. Additionally, always remember to hydrate daily as the blood carries nutrients and oxygen to support immunity and overall health. There are three recipes in the Apothecary section: Oxymel, Immune Tea, and Immune Soup which are excellent ways to support your immune system with food.

Exercise

Remember that exercise plays a positive role in many different body systems including the immune system. Anything that you can do to get moving helps strengthen your body. Yoga has many different kinds to fit your preferences, and might be something to consider when looking for exercises to support immune health. You may want to start with Hatha Yoga as it is more gentle and slow-moving than some of the other variations of yoga. Please refer to Chapters 3-4, 7, 11-14, 16-17, and 19 for more information on exercise, its many benefits, and how to incorporate it into your daily or weekly routine.

Other Therapies to Consider

Hydrotherapy (Constitutional, Contrast, or Heating Compress)

Anytime the immune system must be supported, improved, or modulated, hydrotherapy remains a good option. The most powerful of all the hydrotherapy treatments is constitutional hydrotherapy which is usually done by a practitioner in office or someone's home. If you cannot locate a local practitioner who does constitutional hydrotherapy, consider contrast or heating compress hydrotherapy instead as either can be done by yourself at home. You will get the most benefit from hydrotherapy if you can incorporate it into a weekly practice. Hydrotherapy is discussed in more detail in Chapter 4 and you can find specific instructions in the Apothecary chapter.

Detoxification

Consistent and gentle detoxification with good liver and kidney support is key. See Chapter 8 for a thorough discussion of detoxification.

Chapter 20:
The Apothecary

This chapter provides more details about therapies, recipes, and other information discussed in this book. Nothing listed here is being offered as a treatment suggestion and should be considered purely educational. When items have been listed in a chapter for supporting a particular system, it is not a suggestion to do any particular one nor is it a suggestion to do all of them. Many naturopathic doctors will make recommendations for the specific individual's needs and these needs change from person to person.

Often, a health practitioner will suggest a dosage higher than what is listed on the label in the course of treatment (restoration of health). This is by no means a suggestion for you to do this yourself; instead, it is offered as information to keep in mind that sometimes dosing more than is on the label is appropriate, but should always be monitored by a medical professional. This section contains the basic information for the general population's over-the-counter (OTC) use of various items discussed in this book.

Plant Medicine (Botanicals)

When introducing plant medicine into your daily life, keep in mind some people can have allergic reactions to any new substance including plants. Take things slowly, always try a few drops or a taste of something first. Gradually increase the dose and watch for any symptoms of allergy: rashes, tightness in the chest, difficulty breathing, itching, swelling, etc. If you do develop any of the symptoms mentioned and they persist, seek medical consultation. Also, remember that dosing can vary from one person to the next as well as dosing preferences which can vary from one practitioner to the next.

American Ginseng (*Panax quinquefolius*)

- Part used: root

- Typical use: 1-3 grams of ginseng daily

- It is important to read labels with this one as one of the more active compounds in ginseng, called ginsenosides, can vary in concentration from plant to plant and from product to product. Ginseng is generally well-tolerated, but American ginseng can be overstimulating for some people. If you begin to feel more nervous, edgy, or irritated, this herb may not be the right one for you.

Artichoke (*Cynara cardunculus var. scolymus*)

- Part used: leaf and flower
- Typical use: extract, 300 mg 2-3 times a day
- This can be taken once a day long term to help support liver health, and it is generally well-tolerated. If you are on blood pressure or diabetic medications, please talk with your doctor before introducing this herb into your daily plan.

Ashwagandha (*Withania somnifera*)

- Part used: root
- Typical use: tincture 15-25 ml per day, extract 6-12 ml per day, capsule 600 mg - 2 grams daily in divided doses

Burdock (*Arctium lappa*)

- Part used: Root
- Tea: 1 tsp (5 ml) dried root per 10 oz (285 ml) of water. Place root in a cup, add boiling water and cover, allow to steep for fifteen minutes and strain before drinking. Typical use: 2-4 cups per day, as needed. Optional: sweeten with raw honey and stevia, or add fresh lemon juice

Calendula - see Marigold

Elderberry (*Sambucus nigra*)

- Part used: dried berries
- Tea: 1 tsp (5 ml) dried berries in 10 oz (285 ml) of water. Simmer in a small, covered saucepan for 20 minutes. You will get something that is more medicinal than when pouring boiling water over the berries. Typical use: 2-3 cups of tea a day as needed. Optional: sweeten with raw honey or stevia
- Extract: 1 tsp (5 ml), 2-3 times per day

Dandelion (*Taraxacum officinale*)

- Parts used: leaf (diuretic, mildly stimulating to the liver) and root

(bitter for the digestive system, liver tonic, detoxification support)

- As food: roasted root as a coffee substitute, dandelion wine from flowers and young leaves, as a salad green, juice of pureed leaves
- Tea (root): 2 Tbsp (30 ml) per 10 oz (285 ml) water
- Extract: 1-2 ml, 2-3 times a day

Dark Berry Extracts

- Parts used: Berries
- These are sold as cold-pressed extracts, tinctures, capsules, dried fruits for home brewing, gummies, and likely many other ways. I use cold-pressed extracts and good old-fashioned home brewing with my patients.
- Ideal dose: 1 tsp (5 ml) extract of dark berries 2-3 times a day
- Through diet: add ½ cup (118 ml) of dark berries daily to diet

Ginkgo Biloba

- Part used: leaf
- Tincture: 3-15 ml per day in divided doses
- Fluid Extract: 1-3 ml per day in divided doses
- Infusion: 1 tsp-1 Tbsp (5-15 ml) per 10 oz (285 ml) of water. Place herb in a cup, add boiling water and cover; allow to steep for 5-8 minutes. Cool and strain before drinking.
- Gingko should be dosed for 6 weeks before re-evaluation

Gotu Kola (*Centella asiatica*)

- Part used: whole plant
- Tea: 1-2 tsp (5-10 ml) of herb per 10 oz (285 ml) water, 2-3 times a day
- This can also be used as capsules, 600 mg, three times daily—these doses have been found safe in research studies

Hawthorn (*Crataegus spp.*)

- Part used: Berries, flowers, and leaves
- It can be taken as a tea, tincture, or extract; the solid extract form is preferred
- Infusions (Leaf & Flower): 1 Tbsp (15 ml) per 10 oz (285 ml) water

- Decoctions (Berries): 1 Tbsp (15 ml) per 10 oz (285 ml) water
- Tincture: 60 drops
- Solid Extract: ¼ to ½ tsp (60-120 ml)
- This herb works best if taken more often during the day, 2-3 times a day is recommended
- Generally well tolerated even taking up to 1,800 mg for up to six months' time; most reported side effects are negative gastrointestinal effects, dizziness, and headache

Lavender (*Lavandula angustifolia*)

- Part used: flowers
- Typical use:
  - Tea 1 tsp (5 ml) dried berries in 10 oz (285 ml) of water. Place flowers in a cup, add boiling water and cover; allow to steep for 5-8 minutes. Cool and strain before drinking. Typical use: 2-3 cups of tea a day. Optional: sweeten with a little raw honey or stevia
  - Tincture: 1-3 ml, three times a day
  - Infused Oil: apply topically or use in baths

Lemon balm (*Melissa officinalis*)

- Part used: herbaceous parts
- Lemon balm can be used in food dishes for a nice lemon flavor or as a tea, tincture, or glycerite
- Tinctures and glycerites: 40 drops, 2-3 times a day
- Tea: 1 Tbsp leaves per 10 oz (285 ml) water. Place herb in a cup, add boiling water and cover; allow to steep for 5-8 minutes. Cool and strain before drinking.
- Rarely, lemon balm can cause wheezing; otherwise, it is generally recognized as safe with even higher doses of 3 grams daily being well tolerated

Licorice (*Glycyrrhiza glabra*)

- Part used: root
- Licorice can be used alone as a tea or mixed with other herbs
- Typical dose: between 1 to 3 grams daily. Boil water and pour it

over the herb in a heat-safe mug. Put a cover on the cup, and let it steep for 10 minutes; it takes roots longer to steep than aerial parts of the herb due to the tough outer skin.

- Tincture or glycerite: 40 drops daily
- As this herb is a great synergizer, helping other herbs work better, it is common to see this alongside other herbs in stress formulas
- Again, it is not recommended to use this herb regularly in large doses for long periods of time without guidance from a qualified practitioner. This herb is not recommended for use in those who are pregnant, nursing, or have high blood pressure without first consulting their doctor or a qualified holistic health practitioner. In people who tend to have swelling due to salt intake, this herb should be avoided completely.

Lungwort (*Pulmonaria officinalis*)

- Part used: Leaves
- Tea: 2 tsp (10 ml) of herb per 10 oz (285 ml) of water. Place herb in a cup, add boiling water and cover; allow to steep for 5-8 minutes. Cool and strain before drinking. Typical use: 2-3 cups of tea a day as needed. Some practitioners like to take breaks in using this herb, something like 3 weeks on, 2 weeks off. Optional: sweeten with stevia or raw honey

Marigold (*Calendula officinalis*)

- Part used: Flowers
- Mouthwash: Use 1 Tbsp (15 ml) calendula flowers for 4 oz (120 ml) of water. Add flowers to a mug, pour boiling water, and cover. Allow to steep for 10 minutes, strain the flowers and then rinse your mouth and gargle with the liquid. This should be made fresh each time.
- Topical preparations: there are many to be found, I like calendula ointments
- Poultice applied to the skin

Milk thistle (*Silybum marianum*)

- Part used: leaf and seed
- Preferred forms: The best way to take milk thistle is as a fluid extract or tincture. Supplement quality is generally evaluated by making sure the milk thistle extract is concentrated to at least 70%

silybin. It is safe at higher doses but generally, research supports dosing 240 mg - 900 mg, 2-3 times a day.

- It is recommended to use equal herbs in teas whenever possible. Those who experience some belly upset when consuming milk thistle tea will likely be fine with it as a tincture. As a result, consumption of this herb is recommended in tincture form, though the tea is still a viable option for those who can drink it without discomfort.

Mullein (*Verbascum thapsus*)

- Part used: Leaves
- Mullein is safe to use as long as you are not allergic to it
- Tea: 3 tsp (15 ml) of herb per 10 oz (285 ml) of water. Place herb in a cup, add boiling water and cover; allow to steep for 5-8 minutes. Cool and strain before drinking. Typical use: 2-3 cups of tea a day. Optional: sweeten it with a little raw honey or stevia

Nettle (*Urtica dioica*)

- Part used: herbaceous parts
- Overnight tea: fill a 16 oz (470 ml) glass jar with 2 Tbsp (30 ml) of nettle, fill the remainder with cool, clean water, and let it sit overnight; the next morning, you can start your day with a nourishing herbal drink
- Typical use: 2-3 cups of tea a day as needed. Optional: sweeten it with a little raw honey or stevia

Oat (*Avena sativa*)

- Parts used: milky and mature seeds, straw
- Food: oatmeal as a cereal, bread' a smoothie additive, or cookies (with moderation of course), etc. using oat as a food also increases fiber in your diet, important for daily detoxification
- Tea: use 1 Tbsp (15 ml) milky seeds or straw to 10 oz (285 ml) of water. Place herb in a cup, add boiling water and cover; allow to steep for 5-8 minutes. Cool and strain before drinking. Typical use: 2-3 cups of tea a day. Optional: sweeten with a little raw honey or stevia
- Tincture: 40-60 drops, 2-3 times a day
- Oat is generally considered safe for all populations

Peppermint (*Mentha piperita*)

- Part used: leaf
- Tea: 1-2 tsp (5-10 ml) of herb per 10 oz (285 ml) water, 2-3 times a day
- It can take a week or two before it reaches its maximum potential
- It can be helpful with tonifying and soothing the gastrointestinal tract, but it can cause heartburn as it relaxes the lower esophageal sphincter; thus, avoid this herb if you suffer from heartburn

Red Clover (*Trifolium pratense*)

- Part used: Flowers
- This herb can take some weeks to reach maximal effect, it is typically recommended to take for up to 8 consecutive weeks to see if it is helpful or not
- Research shows isoflavone concentrations from 50-90 mg are most helpful and if you are taking whole herb capsules, you can take 2-3 grams in divided doses in the morning and evening
- If you have a history of breast cancer, make sure you check with your doctor before taking red clover as research is mixed if it is potentially harmful or not

Schisandra (*Schisandra chinensis*)

- Part used: Dried berries
- Typically dosed as an extract of the berries, the dose for this ranges from 1-3 tsp (5-15 ml) 1-3 times a day
- Tea: simmer 1 to 2 Tbsp (15-30 ml) of the dried berries in 16 oz (470 ml) of water in a small, covered saucepan for 20 minutes. You will get something that is more medicinal than when pouring boiling water over the berries. Typical use: 2-3 cups of tea a day as needed. Optional: sweeten with raw honey or stevia
- Just a fun fact, you can do this with elderberries and bilberries as well

Turmeric (*Curcuma longa*)

- Part used: Rhizome (roots)

  Food: use up to 2 grams daily in divided doses (this means taking some in the morning and some in the evening). You can buy turmeric rhizome from your local grocery store depending on where you live. Peel the outside of it with a spoon or peeler. It is absorbed best when eaten with black pepper (*Piper nigrum*) and/or fats. Black pepper alone has been shown to increase turmeric absorption by up to 2,000%. One easy way to add turmeric to your diet is to sprinkle it over eggs in the morning with black pepper; you can cook it in coconut oil, grass-fed butter, etc., which provides the fat component for better absorption.

- Supplement form: capsules, 500-1500 mg per day in divided doses have been used in clinical studies. Extracts carry a more potent action than using turmeric in food. There are times it should be avoided so check with your doctor and visit the Healthline Site at:
  - https://www.healthline.com/nutrition/turmeric-dosage#who-shouldn't-take-it

- One thing to be mindful of is possible lead contamination on the outside of the rhizome or in-ground supplement products. Lead can give tumeric a bright orange color, which is what people often look for in high-quality turmeric. It is strongly recommended to buy organic turmeric or supplements from companies that do quality control testing on their raw ingredients.

Homeopathic Remedies

Building a small home care kit that includes some basic homeopathic remedies is something everyone should take into consideration. Here are two basic 20-remedy kits:

- First Aid Home Kit 30C: Acon, Arn, Apis, Ars, Bell, Bellis, Bry, Canth, Caust, Cocc, Hyper, Ign, Led, Nux v., Phos, Rhus t., Ruta, Staph, Sulph, Urt
- Travel Kit 30C: Acon, Altitude, Arn 30C, Arn 200C, Ars, Bell, Bellis, Cham, Cocc, Con, Cup, Led, Nat-m, Nux v, Ruta, Phos, Puls, Sil, Sulph, Urt-u

This is something you can do for yourself! Under the "Homeopathy" heading of the *Resources* section, you can find some links to wallets and kits. Listed are the ones that hold the typical size remedy sold in health food stores. Or, if you have a homeopathic practitioner, you can check with them and see if they can make you a kit.

Now, what to do with your kit? There are some good basic homeopathic first aid courses out there, many of which are free. It takes just a couple of hours to get started and you can spend a lifetime learning this medicine. There are some good courses listed in the *Resources* section and others listed further on in this chapter.

Specific remedies mentioned in this book include Bryonia, Caladium, Drosera, Hepar sulphuricum, Lobelia inflata, and Nux vomica. Typical dosing is 30C, 3 pellets under the tongue. When you are using potentized medicine for acute or first aid care, dose as needed. If you are considering a homeopathic approach for chronic conditions it is recommended to consult a properly trained homeopathic practitioner.

Nutritional Supplements

Understanding even the very basics about supplements is helpful, especially as you work through creating your own health plan. The quality, source, and preparation of what you take matters. The learning point here is that there are different forms of vitamins, minerals, and other nutritional supplements available on the market shelves. A wholistic health practitioner would be able to evaluate the products you use and often will have their favorite forms and formulations!

CoQ10

For best effect, supplementation should be 100 mg - 200 mg of CoQ10 on a daily basis. As it is a lipid-based antioxidant, it will be best absorbed when taken with food. You can also get additional amounts through your diet. Food sources include oily fish like salmon or sardines, organ meats such as liver or kidney, whole grains, spinach, cauliflower, broccoli, oranges, strawberries, or lentils.

Essential Fatty Acids (EFAs), Fish Oil

If you choose to take supplements, there are dozens of different options out there. Look for fish oil that is molecularly filtered as this will remove the most contaminants, including heavy metals, from the oil. For those who are vegan, you can get algae omega-3 supplements. Generally, taking 2 to 3 grams of fish oil a day is adequate for most people, yet you can take up to 6 grams daily if you tolerate it well. Side effects of high dosing can include loose stools and fish oil burps depending on the fish oil brand you use. A bare minimum for fish oil is 1 teaspoon twice a day (morning and night).

Please note: If you are on blood thinning medications, fish oil may thin your blood further. If you are on this type of medication it is recommended to add no more than 2 grams of fish oil a day, unless you are under a doctor's supervision.

If you'd like to do a more whole food option, eating oily fish twice a week adds an average of 500 mg of omega 3's to your diet. Oily fish includes herring (bloater, kipper, and hilsa are types of herring), pilchards, salmon, sardines, sprats, trout, and mackerel. Whitefish include cod, haddock, plaice, pollock, coley, dab, flounder, red mullet, gurnard, and tilapia which have a lower omega-3 content than oily fish. Some shellfish species are also higher in omega-3s.

For vegans or those who are looking for additional omega-3 sources, you can source omega-3 oils directly from the algae although you'll have to take 2-3 times as much when compared to fish oil; fish eat the algae which contains the omega-3's, which are then concentrated in the fish. Plant sources include seaweed/nori, chia seeds, hemp seeds, flaxseeds, walnuts, edamame, kidney beans, and soybean oil (organic preferred). With soy products, organic is recommended to avoid excess chemical and pesticide exposure. For some ideas on amounts to take, remember 1 tablespoon of flaxseed provides 2.3 grams of omega-3s and 1 tablespoon of chia seed provides 5 grams of omega-3s.

With both of these seeds, it is important to get them in whole form and to store them in the refrigerator to protect the oils in them from becoming rancid. Grind the flaxseeds right before you use them to make the oils easier to absorb in your gut. Flaxseeds can be added to hot cereal, baking recipes, yogurt, smoothies, etc. Chia seeds can also be used in these options, or you can add some milk (almond or coconut tastes best) to them to make chia seed pudding.

Fiber - Psyllium Husk

Remember it's best to get around 30 grams of fiber from your daily diet. Some of the best foods for providing fiber are fruits and vegetables, beans, and whole grains. The best way to get fiber, aside from your diet, is by using a powdered fiber supplement. You can purchase fiber pills, but you'd have to take a handful of them to get enough daily fiber. You can get a powdered psyllium husk supplement which you can add to water, stir, and drink promptly.

Glutathione

Supplementing glutathione can be tricky because it isn't easily absorbed through the gut. The best forms to buy include reduced or liposomal glutathione. Research shows somewhere between 500 to 1000 mg are the best doses to take daily. Foods include asparagus, avocados, okra, and spinach. If you are eating more cruciferous vegetables, make sure you are getting adequate amounts of selenium. Also, eating vitamin C containing foods such as citrus fruits helps keep your glutathione levels higher.

N-acetyl-cysteine (NAC)

Overall research shows taking 600 mg of NAC once or twice a day is effective. The most common side effects included diarrhea, heartburn, and abdominal discomfort though it was well-tolerated at doses above 600 mg. NAC can be taken with food or on its own and it pairs well with vitamin C. For those who have trouble swallowing capsules, mixing the NAC into applesauce, cranberry juice, or peanut butter and honey seems to work well.

Probiotics

Probiotics are best taken with a meal when stomach acid is lower. This will help ensure the microorganisms have a better chance of arriving alive and intact in the intestines. There are many, many different probiotics out there, some shelf-stable, some not. There are probiotics sold over the counter at your local health store which can also be helpful. If you are looking to add this dietarily, you can do this by adding fermented foods into your diet such as sauerkraut, cabbage juice, keifer, yogurt (if dairy is tolerated), pickles, and other pickled vegetables such as kimchi, sourdough bread, natto, etc. For the best effect, it is always recommended to seek advice from a holistic healthcare professional for the best probiotic for your health concerns. Do not use probiotics if you are immune compromised unless you are under the care of a physician.

Hydrotherapy

Contrast Foot Bath

A contrast hydrotherapy foot bath (CHFB) is an excellent way to strengthen your immune system, alleviate congestion, soothe sore muscles, and improve circulation. This hydrotherapy technique involves alternating immersion in cold and hot water for specified times.

- You will need two basins each one large enough for both feet and sufficient water to cover them; fill one basin with ice water, and another with hot water making sure it is not hot enough to cause a burn
- Put your feet in the hot water first for 5 minutes
- Immediately switch to the cold water for 1 minute
- Repeat the process 3-5 times; always ending with the cold water
- Gently dry legs and feet and put on warm socks
- Rest for 20 minutes

Important: if you have inflammation or open wounds on your legs or feet, varicose veins, thrombosis, or phlebitis, consult with your health practitioner before using a contrast foot bath.

Wet Socks

- Just before bed, place a pair of thin, cotton anklets socks in cold water; wring them out well and put them on
- Put on a pair of heavy wool socks that come up over your ankles and climb into bed
- Cover yourself with blankets and sleep all night with the socks on

Heating Compress

Place a large, warm blanket on a bed or couch. You will be wrapping up your body with this. Warm your body first by sitting in the warm sun for 20 minutes or by taking a 15-minute hot bath. Lie down on the blanket and cover your chest and abdomen with a wet, cold, well-wrung-out pillowcase. Wrap up in the blanket. Remain there until the pillow case is dry.

Contrast Hydrotherapy

With a partner, first spread out a thick blanket with a sheet on top of it (wool is preferred but any warm blanket will do on a bed or floor, wherever you are most comfortable). Lay on your back on top of the sheet and blanket near one side. Have your partner take a towel, fold it in half, place the towel in hot water to warm it, then wring it out so it isn't dripping, and cover your torso from your armpits to just above your hips. Your partner can then cover you up with one side of the blanket followed by the other, like a taco. After 5 minutes, replace the hot towel with a cold towel (do not fold) and cover back up in the blanket for 10-15 minutes (until the towel warms up). Next, have your partner repeat this pattern of hot and cold towels on your back. If you are feeling slightly chilled at the end, brush the skin on your back vigorously with a dry towel to warm the area back up.

If you are doing this therapy on yourself, then get the blankets set up as described above. Next, take a hot shower without getting your hair wet. You should feel flushed and/or warm. Dry off quickly, then get a cold towel and wring it out so it isn't dripping water. Wrap this towel around your torso (do not fold it in half, single towel layer only), then cover up in the blankets for 20-30 minutes. If you are cold afterward, rub your skin vigorously with a dry towel. If you are still feeling chilled, get moving by walking or stretching for a few minutes.

Massage and Brushing

Dry Skin Brushing

The use of a dry skin brush is meant to support lymphatic circulation and the removal of old, dead cells from the body. Since lymphatic vessels are superficial, light brushing strokes moving toward the heart are the easiest way to move lymphatic fluid. The lymphatic system does not have its own pump so helping it move either through exercise or dry skin brushing is something that can safely be done by people of all ages.

Lymphatic Massage

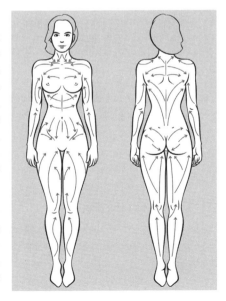

The gentle, soft touch of a lymphatic massage can help remove metabolic waste products and dead cells from the lymphatic system. The information shared through touch extends beyond the physical plane to promote relaxation through interacting with the nervous system. This relaxation helps support the body's efforts to heal itself.

If you are generally healthy, the do-it-yourself version of this technique may be a helpful, inexpensive, at-home therapy. Begin by lightly and gently massaging skin that tops the lymph nodes around your neck, ears, and throat, working the skin along the path of the lymphatic system to help stimulate drainage through the proper channels, then move on to the abdomen and the legs. Starting at the neck will help clear the way for lymph to pump to the lymph nodes as you work on the abdomen and legs. A gentle touch is important because lymphatic vessels are superficial.

Another option is to hire a professional massage therapist or medical practitioner with training in lymphatic drainage massage. Because of the delicate nature of the lymphatic system, and its close proximity to the skin, it is extremely important to work with a professional if you will be using lymphatic massage for a pre-existing condition such as long-term lymphedema, or localized lymphatic swelling.

Lymphatic massage practitioners may be physicians, nurses, physical or occupational therapists, or massage therapists. To find a therapist skilled in lymphatic massage, visit the National Lymphedema Network website, https://lymphnet.org, and be sure to consult your holistic doctor before undergoing treatment to decide if lymphatic massage is a good choice for you.

Abdominal Massage

You can do abdominal massage on bare skin or with lotion. You can even use castor oil topically; just remember, castor oil stains fabric so have an old towel or shirt available. The whole course of the massage follows the large intestine, encouraging stool to move through the intestines. Be careful to follow the instructions mentioned here as the goal is to encourage bowel movements to flow out using a clockwise motion, not back towards the small intestine. Please note this is best done in the evening before bed, but any time of day is fine.

- To begin, lay flat on a bed, a couch, or the floor; use whichever one is most comfortable for you
- Take your hands, one on top of the other, and start from the lower right abdomen and with light but firm pressure move your hands in a small clockwise circle 5 times
- Next, move your hands up about halfway to the top of the abdomen and repeat the clockwise circular motion 5 times
- Continue to massage in small clockwise circles as you move around your abdomen in a larger clockwise circle and end up where you started
- Repeat the entire abdominal massage 5 times

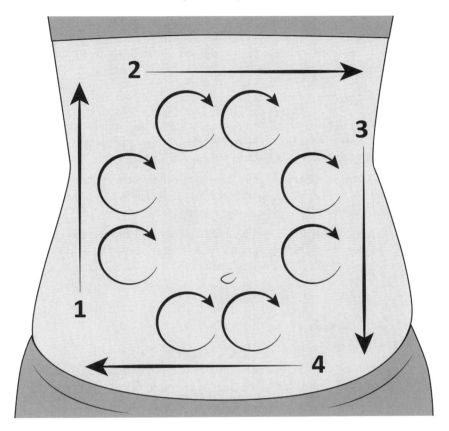

Packs and Compresses

Castor Oil Pack

In order to do this, you need a flannel cloth (cotton or wool is best) that you can fold in half and fit over the treatment area, plastic wrap, a hot water bottle or heating pad, castor oil, and a large food-storage bag. Hot water bottles and castor oil can be found at most pharmacies.

To start, fold the cloth to fit over the treatment area. Put castor oil on the cloth so it is covered in oil, but is not dripping. Lay down in a comfortable position and place the castor oil pack where needed, cover the cloth with plastic wrap, and place the hot water bottle or heating pad over the plastic. Keep the castor oil pack in place for at least 30 minutes, though 60 minutes is ideal to get the maximal effect of the pack. When you are done, place the cloth into the plastic bag. You can use this cloth over and over, adding a little more castor oil when needed. Please note that castor oil stains everything (this is why plastic wrap is recommended), and you may want to have an old towel or rag nearby in case you need to do a little cleanup during or after the therapy.

Alternate Instructions:

- Liver - If you are doing a castor pack over the liver, fold the cloth to fit over your liver which is located in your upper right abdomen with most of it being above your lower ribs
- Abdomen - You can apply the castor oil directly to the abdomen *or* use the castor oil pack; place plastic as needed and follow the rest of the instructions noted above
- Muscle/Joint - This will help with pain—fold the cloth as needed to place over the area; use an ACE wrap if needed to help hold the hot water bottle or heating blanket in place

Mud Pack

- 1-2 teaspoons of clay (bentonite, French green, etc.)
- 1-2 teaspoons of water (use more if needed)
- 1-2 teaspoons additional additives you can consider such as raw honey or powdered herbs such as plantain, calendula, aloe, etc.
- Add the powders together first and mix, then add honey, aloe vera gel, or other liquids and stir it into a thick paste
- Add water, a little at a time, until the paste thins out
- Apply the paste to the face or other parts of the body in gentle circular motions; avoid the eyes, nostrils, and mouth
- Let the pack sit on the skin until hardened (roughly 15 minutes or so), then remove with a damp washcloth
- Gently pat your skin dry with a towel

Recipes

Bieler's Broth

This recipe is an alkalizing formula that promotes pH balancing.

Ingredients:

- 2 medium zucchini, chopped
- Handful of fresh green beans
- 2 stalks of celery, chopped
- 2 potatoes, unpeeled, chopped
- 1 cup chopped carrots
- 1 cup any other available dark green vegetable (collards, chard, kale, etc.)
- 1 cup tops (beets, turnips, radishes, etc.)
- 1 and ½ quarts of water

Directions:

- Boil zucchini, green beans, celery, potatoes, carrots, dark green vegetables, and tops in a covered pot until very soft
- Add cayenne, basil, oregano, and other desired seasonings, except salt. Cover and cook slowly for 1-2 hours; cool for 30 minutes, strain and drink only the broth, 2 cups a day

Immune Tea (The Elder Tea)

This recipe- makes 2 ¼ cups of loose tea

Ingredients:

- 1 (240 ml) cup lemon balm (leaves)
- 1 cup (240 ml) oat straw (chopped straw)
- 1/4 cup (60 ml) astragalus root, minced or chopped
- 1/4 cup (60 ml) elderberry (dried berries)
- 1/4 cup (60 ml) rose hips (flowers)
- 1/4 cup (60 ml) hibiscus (flowers)

- 1/8 cup (30 ml) licorice root, minced or chopped
- 1/8 cup (30 ml) ginger root, minced or chopped

Directions:

- Mix all herbs in a large container; store in a dry, airtight container
- To make a cup of tea: use 2 Tbsp (30 ml) of herb blend per 10 oz (285 ml) of water. Place in a small pot with a lid and simmer for 15 minutes. Let cool for 2 min, strain, and drink; sweeten with a little honey or stevia and a squeeze of fresh lemon, and enjoy warm or cold

Immune Soup

This is a yummy and nutritious pot of goodness!

Ingredients:

- You will need a "make it yourself" large tea bag or some cheesecloth to contain the Astragalus and Reishi mushroom
- 8 cups (1.9 liters) water
- 1 tablespoon (15 ml) sunflower oil
- 1 medium onion, diced
- 1 bulb garlic (at least 10 cloves), minced
- 1 and 1/2 inch (3 and 1/2 cm) piece of fresh ginger root, finely grated
- 2 stalks celery, chopped
- 5 pieces sliced dried astragalus root
- 1 large reishi mushroom
- 2 cups (475 ml) fresh, sliced shiitake mushrooms
- 2 cups (475 ml) chopped kale
- 2 medium carrots, chopped
- ½ tsp (2.5 ml) cayenne powder
- 1 tsp (5 ml) salt (to taste)
- 1 tsp (5 ml) black pepper
- ½ tsp (2.5 ml) miso (optional)

Directions:

- Put astragalus root and reishi mushroom in a large self-sealing tea bag or cheesecloth tied at the top
- Bring water to boil in a large pot
- While water is coming to a boil, add the astragalus and reishi bag, reduce to a simmer and cook covered for 2 hours
- Add all remaining ingredients except cayenne, salt, pepper, and miso
- Return to a boil and then reduce to simmer; cook for 30 min
- Remove from heat and allow to sit covered until served
- Before serving, remove the astragalus and reishi bag and discard; add salt, pepper and cayenne, and adjust to taste; you can also add miso if desired

Oxymel, Garlic, and Ginger

Ingredients:

- 1 bulb garlic
- 1 Tbsp (30 ml) finely minced fresh ginger root
- 4 cups water (1 liter)
- ¼ cup raw honey (60 ml)
- ¼ cup apple cider vinegar (60 ml)

Directions:

- Peel and finely chop garlic cloves. Do not use the pre-peeled and minced garlic sold in stores as this has already begun oxidizing
- Place the garlic in a large pot filled with water and cover, heat to boiling. Boil until the garlic is very soft, about 20 minutes
- Remove from heat and allow to cool for at least 1 hour
- Add honey and vinegar, mix well
- Store in the refrigerator for up to 5 days and gently reheat on the stove before drinking. ½ - 1 cup (120 - 240 ml) per day

A Smoker's Daily Plan

Now that you have been introduced to all the different systems, and read chapters on creating health in general, you might feel a bit overwhelmed. After all, if you do everything in every chapter, you will be doing nothing but attending to your health most of the day! This chapter brings everything together with a few different approaches for a daily plan without having to take 30 supplements a day or make hundreds of changes all at one time.

If there is a system in your body that seems to be struggling, for example, perhaps you have significant respiratory issues, take your Daily Plan and add to it from the Respiratory System Chapter. There will be overlap between that chapter and others in various things, but there is no need to double up in your daily plan. For example, in supplements, the only additional one you would consider is NAC. From the Botanical section you would pick one of the herbs, but not all of them. You might also consider adding selenium-rich foods and dark berries to your diet or picking a breathing exercise to incorporate into your everyday routine.

Always remember to check in with your holistic practitioner before beginning any major dietary, exercise, or supplement regime.

Basic General Plan

Here is a general daily plan to help elevate the health of a smoker. Start small, make the change a part of your everyday life, and when you have incorporated that change successfully, move on to the next one. Even if it takes you three years to shift into living a healthier life, it is worth it in the long run.

Diet

- Eat a whole foods diet as much as possible
- Eat 7 colorful fruits and/ or vegetables each day, especially dark leafy greens
- Include fiber in your diet from vegetables and whole grains
- Eat plant fats primarily and animal fats sparingly
- Consume red meat sparingly and eat abundantly of fruits, grains, nuts, seeds, and veggies

- Eat a variety of foods
- Limit sugar intake to occasional treats
- Decrease or eliminate all known food sensitivities/allergens; if you are not sure, consider having a food allergy blood test done
- Use a vitamin and mineral supplement as suggested by your practitioner
- Revisit chapters 3 and 4 as needed to develop your diet plan

Drink

- Consume plenty of fresh filtered water daily. A general starting point is to drink ½ your body weight in ounces. This must be individualized based on your diet and activity, medications, and general health status. Example: weight = 200 pounds then divide in half to get 100 ounces per day
- Use a water filter depending on the quality of your water
- Limit or eliminate caffeine consumption
- Decrease or eliminate soda and other sugary drinks
- Revisit Chapter 3

Exercise

- Have a physical before starting any new exercise program
- Incorporate at least 30 minutes of regular exercise three to four times a week
- Add cardio and resistance training as you are able, 2 times a week
- Walk everywhere you can
- Stretch every day
- Breath deeply on a regular basis
- Chapters 3-4, 7, 11-14, and 16-18

Sleep

- Get 7-10 hours of sleep each night
- Schedule time to prepare, relax, fall asleep, stretch, and wake up

- Stop evening activities (screentime) at least 1 hour before you need to be asleep
- Eliminate caffeine (if you haven't already) in the afternoon
- Chapters 3-4 and 18

Environmental Considerations

- Use air and water filters
- Purchase only organic thin-skinned fruits and vegetables
- Avoid cooking and drinking out of plastic containers
- Grow a plant or two in your indoor spaces
- Visit the Environmental Working Group's website, www.ewg.org, and use the lists they produce to avoid many toxins
- Read labels

Core Supplements

- Multiple vitamin and mineral
- Trace minerals in addition to the minerals in your multiple vitamin
- EFAs
- Vitamin C in addition to what is in your multiple vitamin
- Magnesium in addition to what is in your multiple vitamin
- Glutathione
- CoQ10
- Reminder: make sure to read labels to avoid getting too much of a good thing
- Supplements are discussed in every chapter, but for a more in-depth discussion see Chapters 3 and 4

Core Therapies

- Hydrotherapy (discussed throughout the book, Chapter 4, Apothecary)
- Castor oil packs (Chapters 3 and 8, Apothecary)

- Stress relief (discussed throughout the book, Chapter 12)
- Regular detoxification (Chapter 8)
- Deep breathing practice (Chapters 6 and 7)

Closing Thoughts

There is a key concept that runs throughout this book. Symptoms are not something to be treated. Symptoms are clues that reveal how the body is unbalanced and where health needs to be restored.

It is the person that needs to be treated so their body can heal itself.

There has been more than enough research done on how to be healthy, how not, and what it means to be in one state or the other. Most doctors, healers, and especially scientists will readily agree that a body less than healthy enough will show symptoms indicating there is something more going on.

Those in the medical profession call that something illness.

And those same professionals will also agree that a body in a healthy state, functioning as it should, will not show symptoms of illness, because it isn't ill.

This is when folks have reached a level of being healthy enough.

The job of the doctor, the healer, is to teach people what to do, what not to do, and how to help their body restore health as much as possible so there is no need for symptoms of illness.

You or someone you love is a smoker. You know, I know, they know, that the best thing they can do is to quit smoking. But, if you accept the choice to smoke, what then? Well, the next best thing is to use the information in this book to create a healthier body.

Thanks for reading. I would be honored if you would tell everyone you know about this book. Then we can help as many people as possible do something, anything, that leaves them in a more healthful state.

E Camp, ND, DHANP
Aug 2022

Resources

Homeopathy

- HOMÉOPATHE INTERNATIONAL is an organization which provides access to many different kinds of homeopathic resources; membership is not required but there is a voluntary option for membership: http://homeoint.org/english/index.htm
- Whole Health Now: http://www.wholehealthnow.com/
- Homeopathic Educational: https://www.homeopathic.com/
- For a basic understanding of Homeopathy, Beyond Flat Earth Medicine by Dr. Dooley, http://www.drdooley.net/Book.pdf
- Homeopathy Research Institute lists current research and completed projects: https://www.hri-research.org/hri-research/
- The Canadian Academy of Homeopathy Research and Development: https://www.homeopathy.ca/research-development/
- Wallets and kits:
    - Remedia wallets (that hold the size from the health shop, 1 ml tubes): https://www.remedia-homeopathy.com/shop/Leather-Cases/c313?searchTerm=&facet-Type+of+case=remedia+tubes
    - Storage boxes from MTM Medical: http://www.mtmmedical.com/hingedvialstorageboxes.html
    - Kits from Washington Homeopathic: https://www.homeopathyworks.com/30c-200c-homeopathic-remedy-kit

Plant Medicine

- A wonderful guide to plant medicine from James Green, *The Herbal Medicine-Makers' Handbook: A Home Manual*
- Rosemary Gladstar wrote *Medicinal Herbs: A Beginner's Guide: 33 Healing Herbs to Know, Grow, and Use* is an excellent place to start
- If you are interested in taking a course, The Herbal Academy is an excellent place to learn: https://theherbalacademy.com/herbalism-courses/

Nutrition

- Cronometer—an excellent way to check your nutrition: https://cronometer.com/
- Oxford Home Study Center, free online nutrition training, great for beginners: https://www.oxfordhomestudy.com/courses/nutrition-certificate-programs-online/free-online-nutrition-courses
- edX free nutrition courses: https://www.edx.org/learn/nutrition
- *The Academy of Nutrition and Dietetics Complete Food and Nutrition Guide*, by Roberta Larson Duyff
- *Eat, Drink, and Be Healthy: The Harvard Medical School Guide to Eating*

Kicking the Habit

For help with kicking the habit, here are a few helpful resources.

- Smoke Free: https://smokefree.gov/
- From the American Lung Association, I Want to Quit: https://www.lung.org/quit-smoking/i-want-to-quit
- CDC 7 Common Withdrawal Symptoms and What to Do: https://www.cdc.gov/tobacco/campaign/tips/quit-smoking/7-common-withdrawal-symptoms/index.html
- From Cancer.net, a comprehensive list of associations and organization with contact information: https://www.cancer.net/navigating-cancer-care/prevention-and-healthy-living/stopping-tobacco-use-after-cancer-diagnosis/resources-help-you-quit-smoking
- If you can get this paper from your local university or public library, it discusses many of the alternative medicine approaches:Amit Sood, M.D., M.Sc., Jon O. Ebbert, M.D., M.Sc., Richa Sood, M.D., Susanna R. Stevens, B.S., "Complementary Treatments for Tobacco Cessation: A Survey," *Nicotine and Tobacco Research*, Volume 8, Issue 6, December 2006, Pages 767–771, https://doi. org/10.1080/14622200601004109
- My favorite book to recommend to people who want to explore quitting is Allen Carr's *Easy Way to Stop Smoking*

References

Abarikwu, S. O., C. L. Onuah, and S. K. Singh. 2020. *Plants in the Management of Male Infertility. Andrologia, 52(3).* doi:10.1111/and.13509.

Abbasi, Behnood, et al. 2012. "The Effect of Magnesium Supplementation on Primary Insomnia in Elderly: A Double-Blind Placebo-Controlled Clinical Trial." *Journal of Research in Medical Sciences: The Official Journal of Isfahan University of Medical Sciences,* 17(12): 1161-9.

Acupuncture One: von Trott, Philipp, et al. 2020. "Acupuncture for Breathlessness in Advanced Diseases: A Systematic Review and Meta-analysis." *Journal of pain and symptom management,* 59(2): 327-338. e3. doi:10.1016/j.jpainsymman.2019.09.007.

Adhikari, Bhaskar Mani, et al. 2015. "Comparison of Nutritional Properties of Stinging Nettle (Urtica dioica) Flour With Wheat and Barley Flours." *Food Science and Nutrition,* 4(1): 119-24. doi:10.1002/fsn3.259.

Ahmad, Rabia Shabir, et al. 2020. "Biochemistry, Safety, Pharmacological Activities, and Clinical Applications of Turmeric: A Mechanistic Review." *Evidence-Based Complementary and Alternative Medicine: eCAM,* 2020: 7656919. doi:10.1155/2020/7656919.

Ahmadi-Motamayel, Fatemeh, et al. 2016. "Comparison of Salivary pH, Buffering Capacity and Alkaline Phosphatase in Smokers and Healthy Non-Smokers: Retrospective Cohort Study." *Sultan Qaboos University Medical Journal,* 16(3): e317-21. doi:10.18295/squmj.2016.16.03.009.

Alam, Iftikhar, et al. 2019. "Recurrent Circadian Fasting (RCF) Improves Blood Pressure, Biomarkers Of Cardiometabolic Risk and Regulates Inflammation in Men." *Journal of Translational Medicine,* 17(1): 272. doi:10.1186/s12967-019-2007-z.

Alam, Murad, et al. 2018. "Association of Facial Exercise With the Appearance of Aging." *JAMA dermatology,* 154(3): 365-367. doi:10.1001/jamadermatol.2017.5142.

Alammar, N., et al. 2019. "The Impact Of Peppermint Oil on The Irritable Bowel Syndrome: A Meta-Analysis of the Pooled Clinical Data". *BMC Complementary and Alternative Medicine,* 19(1): 21. doi:10.1186/s12906-018-2409-0.

Al-Bashaireh, Ahmad M., et al. 2018. "The Effect of Tobacco Smoking on Musculoskeletal Health: A Systematic Review." *Journal of Environmental and Public Health,* 2018: 4184190. doi:10.1155/2018/4184190.

Allen, H. C. 1978. *Keynotes and Characteristics With Comparisons of Some of the Leading Remedies of the Materia Medica.* Thorsons.

Almario, Christopher V., et al. 2018. "Burden of Gastrointestinal Symptoms in the United States: Results of a Nationally Representative Survey of Over 71,000 Americans." *The American Journal of Gastroenterology,* 113(11): 1701-1710. doi:10.1038/s41395-018-0256-8.

Alpha-Tocopherol, Beta Carotene Cancer Prevention Study Group. 1994. "The Effect Of Vitamin E And Beta Carotene On The Incidence Of Lung Cancer And Other Cancers In Male Smokers." *The New England Journal Of Medicine,* 330(15): 1029-35. doi:10.1056/NEJM199404143301501.

Al-Snafi, Ali. 2015. "The Nutritional and Therapeutic Importance of Avena Sativa - An Overview". *International Journal of Phytotherapy,* 5: 48-56.

Alwis, K. Udeni, et al. 2015. "Acrolein Exposure in U.S. Tobacco Smokers and Non-

Tobacco Users: NHANES 2005-2006." *Environmental health perspectives*, 123(12): 1302-8. doi:10.1289/ehp.1409251.

Aly, Eman Mohamed, and Mervat Ahmed Ali. n.d. "Effects of Bilberry on Deoxyribonucleic Acid damage and Oxidant-Antioxidant Balance in the Lens, Induced by Ultraviolet Radiation." *The Malaysian Journal of Medical Sciences: MJMS*, 21(1): 11-8.

American Lung Association. n.d. "Toxic Air Pollutants." Accessed Dec. 19, 2021. https://www.lung.org/clean-air/outdoors/what-makes-air-unhealthy/toxic-air-pollutants.

American Lung Society. n.d. "Breathing Exercises." Accessed Nov. 28, 2021. https://www.lung.org/lung-health-diseases/wellness/breathing-exercises.

American Society for Nutrition. n.d. "Most Americans Are Not Getting Enough Fiber in Our Diets." Last modified June 9, 2021. https://nutrition.org/most-americans-are-not-getting-enough-fiber-in-our-diets/.

Anderson, R. A., et al. 1997. "Elevated Intakes of Supplemental Chromium Improve Glucose and Insulin Variables in Individuals With Type 2 Diabetes." *Diabetes*, 46(11): 1786-91. doi:10.2337/diab.46.11.1786.

Ansary, J., T. Y. Forbes-Hernández, E. Gil, D. Cianciosi, J. Zhang, M. Elexpuru-Zabaleta, J. Simal-Gandara, F. Giampieri, and M. Battino. 2020. "Potential Health Benefit of Garlic Based on Human Intervention Studies: A Brief Overview". Basel, Switzerland: *Antioxidants*, 9(7): 619. https://doi.org/10.3390/antiox9070619.

Arias, I. M. and H. J. Alter. 2009. *The Liver: Biology and Pathobiology*, 5th ed. Wiley-Blackwell.

Arnaud Chiolero, David Faeh, Fred Paccaud, Jacques Cornuz. 2008. "Consequences of Smoking for Body Weight, Body Fat Distribution, and Insulin Resistance". *The American Journal of Clinical Nutrition*, 87(4): 801–809. https://doi.org/10.1093/ajcn/87.4.801.

Arosio, Beatrice, and Matteo Cesari. 2021. "Nutrition and Muscle Health." *Nutrients*, 13(3): 797. doi:10.3390/nu13030797.

Ask The Scientists. n.d. "Liver Detoxification Pathways." Accessed January 7, 2022. https://askthescientists.com/qa/liver-detoxification-pathways/.

Asl, Marjan Nassiri, and Hossein Hosseinzadeh. 2008. "Review of Pharmacological Effects of Glycyrrhiza sp. and Its Bioactive Compounds." *Phytotherapy Research: PTR*, 22(6): 709-24. doi:10.1002/ptr.2362.

Avis-Riiordan, Katie. n.d. "Ginkgo Biloba: The Tree that Outlived the Dinosaurs". Reviewed May 5, 2020. https://www.kew.org/read-and-watch/ginkgo-biloba-maidenhair-tree-kew-gardens.

Babiker, Amir, et al. 2020. "The Role of Micronutrients in Thyroid Dysfunction." *Sudanese Journal of Pediatrics*, 20(1): 13-19. doi:10.24911/SJP.106-1587138942.

Badrick, E., C. Kirschbaum, and M. Kumari. 2007. "The Relationship Between Smoking Status and Cortisol Secretion." *The Journal of Clinical Endocrinology and Metabolism*, 92(3): 819–824. doi:10.1210/jc.2006-2155.

Baillie-Hamilton, P. 2005. *Stop the 21st Century Killing You: Toxic Chemicals Have Invaded Our Lives*. Vermilion.

Balch, P. A. and J. F. Balch. 1992-1987. *Rx Prescription for Cooking and Dietary Wellness*, revised. P. A. B. Pub.

Baltaci, Abdulkerim Kasim, et al. 2019. "Review: The Role of Zinc in the Endocrine System." *Pakistan Journal of Pharmaceutical Sciences*, 32(1): 231-239.

Bansal A., A. Kaushik, C. M. Singh, V. Sharma, H. Singh. 2015. "The Effect of Regular Physical Exercise on the Thyroid Function of Treated Hypothyroid Patients: An Interventional Study at a Tertiary Care Center in Bastar Region of India". *Arch Med Health Sci.*, 3: 244-6.

Barroso, Marina Valente, et al. 2017. "Propolis Reversed Cigarette Smoke-Induced Emphysema Through Macrophage Alternative Activation Independent of Nrf2." *Bioorganic and Medicinal Chemistry*, 25(20): 5557-5568. doi:10.1016/j.bmc.2017.08.026.

Bazzini, Claudia, et al. 2013. "Short-and Long-Term Effects of Cigarette Smoke Exposure on Glutathione Homeostasis in Human Bronchial Epithelial Cells." *Cellular Physiology and Biochemistry: International Journal of Experimental Cellular Physiology, Biochemistry, and Pharmacology*, 32(7): 129-45. doi:10.1159/000356633.

Bede, O., et al. n.d. "Effects of Magnesium Supplementation on the Glutathione Redox System in Atopic Asthmatic Children." *Inflammation Research: Official Journal of the European Histamine Research Society*, 57(6): 279-86. doi:10.1007/s00011-007-7077-3.

Berlin, I. 2009. "Endocrine and Metabolic Effects of Smoking Cessation". *Current Medical Research and Opinion*, 25(2): 527–534. doi:10.1185/03007990802707626.

Better Health Channel. n.d. "Metabolism". Reviewed April 30, 2020. https://www.betterhealth.vic.gov.au/health/conditionsandtreatments/metabolism.

Blanco-Salas, José, et al. 2021. "Searching for Scientific Explanations for the Uses of Spanish Folk Medicine: A Review on the Case of Mullein (Verbascum, Scrophulariaceae)." *Biology*, 10(7): 618. doi:10.3390/biology10070618.

Boericke, William. n.d. *Homoeopathic Materia Medica*. Accessed January 5, 2022. http://www.homeoint.org/books/boericmm/.

Boksa, Patricia. 2017. "Smoking, Psychiatric Illness and the Brain." *Journal of Psychiatry and Neuroscience: JPN*, 42(3): 147-149. doi:10.1503/jpn.170060.

Booth, N. L., C. E. Piersen, S. Banuvar, S. E. Geller, L. P. Shulman, and N. R. Farnsworth. 2006. "Clinical Studies of Red l(Trifolium Pratense) Dietary Supplements in Menopause: a Literature Review". *Menopause*, 13(2): 251–264. doi:10.1097/01.gme.0000198297.

Booth, Nancy L., et al. 2006. "Clinical Studies of Red Clover (Trifolium Pratense) Dietary Supplements in Menopause: A Literature Review." New York: *Menopause*, 13(2): 251-64. doi:10.1097/01.gme.0000198297.40269.f7.

Boyle, W. and Saine André. 1988. *Lectures in Naturopathic Hydrotherapy*. Buckeye Naturopathic Press.

Bradberry, J. Chris, and Daniel E. Hilleman. 2013. "Overview of Omega-3 Fatty Acid Therapies." *P and T : A Peer-Reviewed Journal for Formulary Management*, 38(11): 681-91.

Breus, Michael. "Physical Health." n.d. The Sleep Doctor. Accessed Sept. 27, 2022. https://thesleepdoctor.com/physical-health/

Buscemi, Silvio, et al. 2018. "The Effect of Lutein on Eye and Extra-Eye Health." *Nutrients*, 10(9): 1321. doi:10.3390/nu10091321.

Calderón-Ospina, Carlos Alberto, and Mauricio Orlando Nava-Mesa. 2020. "B Vitamins in the Nervous System: Current Knowledge of The Biochemical Modes of Action and Synergies of Thiamine, Pyridoxine, and Cobalamin." *CNS Neuroscience and Therapeutics*, 26(1): 5-13. doi:10.1111/cns.13207.

Calverley, Peter, et al. 2021. "Safety of N-Acetylcysteine at High Doses in Chronic Respiratory Diseases: A Review." *Drug safety*, 44(3): 273-290. doi:10.1007/s40264-020-01026-y.

Camfield, David A., et al. 2013. "The Effects of Multivitamin Supplementation on Diurnal Cortisol Secretion and Perceived Stress." *Nutrients*, 5(11): 4429-50. doi:10.3390/nu5114429.

Cannon W. B. and L. B. Nice. 1913. *The Effect of Adrenal Secretion on Muscular Fatigue*. Plimpton Press.

Caputo, M., et al. 2020. "Inositols and Metabolic Disorders: From Farm to Bedside." *Journal of Traditional and Complementary Medicine*, 10(3): 252-259. doi:10.1016/j.jtcme.2020.03.005.

Carr, Anitra C., and Silvia Maggini. 2017. "Vitamin C and Immune Function." *Nutrients*, 9(11): 1211. doi:10.3390/nu9111211.

Castañeda, R., S. Natarajan, S. Y. Jeong, B. N. Hong, and T. H. Kang. 2018. "Traditional Oriental Medicine for Sensorineural Hearing Loss: Can Ethnopharmacology Contribute to Potential Drug Discovery?". *Journal of Ethnopharmacology*. doi:10.1016/j.jep.2018.11.016.

CDCTobaccoFree. 2021. "Youth and Tobacco Use." *Centers for Disease Control and Prevention*, April 22, 2021. https://www.cdc.gov/tobacco/data_statistics/fact_sheets/youth_data/tobacco_use/index.htm.

Çelik, Sercan Bulut, et al. 2017. "Evaluation of The Neuropathic Pain in the Smokers." *Agri: Agri (Algoloji) Dernegi'nin Yayin Organidir = The Journal of the Turkish Society of Algology*, 29(3): 122-126. doi:10.5505/agri.2017.68815.

Center for Disease Control. n.d. "Benefits of Physical Activity." Accessed November 11, 2021. https://www.cdc.gov/physicalactivity/basics/pa-health/index.htm.

Center for Disease Control and Prevention. n.d. "Sodium." Accessed Dec. 15, 2020. https://www.cdc.gov/heartdisease/sodium.htm.

Centers for Disease Control and Prevention (US); National Center for Chronic Disease Prevention and Health Promotion (US); Office on Smoking and Health (US). 2010. "How Tobacco Smoke Causes Disease: The Biology and Behavioral Basis for Smoking-Attributable Disease: A Report of the Surgeon General." Atlanta: *Centers for Disease Control and Prevention (US)*. https://www.ncbi.nlm.nih.gov/books/NBK53021/.

Chan, Y. S., L. N. Cheng, J. H. Wu, E. Chan, Y. W. Kwan, S. M. Y. Lee, ... S. W. Chan. 2010. *A Review of the Pharmacological Effects of Arctium Lappa (Burdock)*. *Inflammopharmacology*, 19(5), 245–254. doi:10.1007/s10787-010-0062-4.

Chang, Jiwon, et al. 2016. "Effect of Cigarette Smoking and Passive Smoking on Hearing Impairment: Data from a Population-Based Study." *PloS One*, 11(1): e0146608. doi:10.1371/journal.pone.0146608.

Chao, Limin, et al. 2020. "Effects of Probiotics on Depressive or Anxiety Variables in Healthy Participants Under Stress Conditions or With a Depressive or Anxiety Diagnosis: A Meta-Analysis of Randomized Controlled Trials." *Frontiers in Neurology*, 11: 421. doi:10.3389/fneur.2020.00421.

Chaput, Jean-Philippe, et al. 2018. "Sleeping hours: What is the Ideal Number and How Does Age Impact This?". *Nature and Science of Sleep*, Nov. 27, 2018, 10: 421-430. doi:10.2147/NSS.S163071.

Chen, Xia, et al. 2014. "Antioxidant and Anti-Inflammatory Effects of *Schisandra* and *Paeonia* Extracts in the Treatment of Asthma." *Experimental And Therapeutic Medicine*, 8(5): 1479-1483. doi:10.3892/etm.2014.1948.

Chéruel, Fabrice, et al. 2017. "Effect of Cigarette Smoke on Gustatory Sensitivity, Evaluation of the Deficit and of the Recovery Time-Course After Smoking Cessation." *Tobacco Induced Diseases*, 15: doi:10.1186/s12971-017-0120-4.

Choi, Ga-Ya, et al. n.d. "Effects of Panax Ginseng on the Sperm Motility and Spermatogenesis in the SD Rat." *Korean Journal of Oriental Medicine*, 25(4): 90-94. https://www.jkom.org/upload/10-Effects%20of%20Panax%20Ginseng%20

on(105558).PDF.

Choi, So Hee, Hamidovic Ajna. 2020. "Association Between Smoking and Premenstrual Syndrome: A Meta-Analysis." *Frontiers in Psychiatry*, 11. https://www.frontiersin.org/article/10.3389/fpsyt.2020.575526.

Chrubasik, Julia E., et al. 2007. "A Comprehensive Review on the Stinging Nettle Effect and Efficacy Profiles. Part II: Urticae Radix." *Phytomedicine: International Journal of Phytotherapy and Phytopharmacology*, 14(7-8): 568-79. doi:10.1016/j.phymed.2007.03.014.

Clarke, John Henry. n.d. *Materia Medica*. Accessed January 5, 2022. https://www.materiamedica.info/en/materia-medica/john-henry-clarke/index.

Cleveland Clinic. n.d. "Diaphragmatic Breathing." Reviewed Sept. 14, 2018. https://my.clevelandclinic.org/health/articles/9445-diaphragmatic-breathing.

Clifford, Tom, et al. 2015. "The Potential Benefits of Red Beetroot Supplementation in Health And Disease." *Nutrients*, 7(4): 2801-22. doi:10.3390/nu7042801.

Cohen, Marc Maurice. 2014. "Tulsi - Ocimum Sanctum: A Herb for All Reasons." *Journal of Ayurveda and Integrative Medicine*, 5(4): 251-9. doi:10.4103/0975-9476.146554.

Cooper, Jeffery. n.d. "Summary of Research on the Efficacy of Vision Therapy for Specific Visual Dysfunctions". Accessed May 26, 2022. https://www.neurovisualperformance.ca/education/research-papers/summary-of-research-on-the-efficacy-of-vision-therapy-for-specific-visual-dysfunctions/.

Coulston, A. M., C. Boushey, and M. G. Ferruzzi. 2013. *Nutrition in the Prevention and Treatment of Disease*, 3rd ed. Elsevier/Academic.

Cowell, Whitney et al. 2017. "Ground Turmeric as a Source of Lead Exposure in the United States." *Public Health Reports (Washington, D.C.: 1974)*, 132(3): 289-293. doi:10.1177/0033354917700109.

Crinnion, W. 2010. *Clean Green and Lean: Get Rid of the Toxins That Make You Fat*. John Wiley.

Crinnion, W. J. 2010. "Organic Foods Contain Higher Levels of Certain Nutrients, Lower Levels of Pesticides and May Provide Health Benefits for the Consumer." *Alternative Medicine Review: A Journal of Clinical Therapeutic*: 4-12.

Cronkleton, Emily. 2021. "Can Face Yoga Improve Your Appearance?" *Healthline*, Feb. 11, 2021. https://www.healthline.com/health/fitness-exercise/face-yoga#exercises.

Cronkleton, Emily. n.d. "Yoga for Thyroid." Reviewed July 12, 2017. https://www.healthline.com/health/yoga-for-thyroid.

Culpeper, N. 1858. *Culpeper's Complete Herbal: With Nearly Four Hundred Medicines Made From English Herbs Physically Applied to the Cure Of All Disorders Incident to Man With Rules for Compounding Them Also Directions for Making Syrups Ointments &c. &c. &c.* Milner and Sowerby. Accessed Aug. 29, 2022. http://books.google.com/books?id=jZcyAQAAMAAJ.

Dai, Hongjian, et al. 2021. "Dietary Hawthorn-Leaves Flavonoids Improves Ovarian Function and Liver Lipid Metabolism in Aged Breeder Hens." *Poultry Science*, 100(12): 101499. doi:10.1016/j.psj.2021.101499.

Dallongeville, Jean, Nadine Marécaux, Jean-Charles Fruchart, Philippe Amouyel. 1998. "Cigarette Smoking Is Associated with Unhealthy Patterns of Nutrient Intake: a Meta-Analysis". *The Journal of Nutrition*, 128(9): 1450–1457, https://doi.org/10.1093/jn/128.9.1450.

Dalvi, S. 2003. *Adrenal Fatigue: A Desk Reference*. Authors OnLine.

Daniele, C., G. Mazzanti, M. H. Pittler, and E. Ernst. 2006. *Adverse-Event Profile of*

Crataegus Spp. *Drug Safety, 29(6): 523–535.* doi:10.2165/00002018-200629060.

Darabseh, M. Z.., T. M. Maden-Wilkinson, G. Welbourne, et al. 2021. "Fourteen Days Of Smoking Cessation Improves Muscle Fatigue Resistance and Reverses Markers Of Systemic Inflammation". *Sci Rep*, 11: 12286. https://doi.org/10.1038/s41598-021-91510-x.

Davis, D. R., M. D. Epp, and H D. Riordan. 2004. "Changes in USDA Food Composition Data for 43 Garden Crops, 1950 to 1999." *Journal of the American College of Nutrition, 23(6): 669–682.* https://doi.org/10.1080/07315724.2004.10719409.

Davis, E. A., and D. J. Morris. 1991. "Medicinal Uses of Licorice Through the Millennia: The Good and Plenty of it". *Molecular and Cellular Endocrinology, 78(1-2): 1–6.* doi:10.1016/0303-7207(91)90179-v.

De Angelis, Cristina, et al. 2020. "Smoke, Alcohol and Drug Addiction and Female Fertility." *Reproductive Biology and Endocrinology: RB&E*, 18(1): 21. doi:10.1186/s12958-020-0567-7.

De Cabo, R., and M. P. Mattson. 2019. *Effects of Intermittent Fasting on Health, Aging, and Disease. New England Journal of Medicine, 381(26), 2541–2551.* doi:10.1056/nejmra1905136.

Del Bo', C., M. Porrini, D. Fracassetti, J. Campolo, D. Klimis-Zacas, and P. Riso. 2014. "A Single Serving of Blueberry (V. Corymbosum) Modulates Peripheral Arterial Dysfunction Induced by Acute Cigarette Smoking in Young Volunteers: A Randomized-Controlled Trial". *Food Funct.*, 5(12): 3107–3116. doi:10.1039/c4fo00570h.

De Souza Predes, Fabricia, et al. 2014. "Hepatoprotective effect of Arctium lappa root extract on cadmium toxicity in adult Wistar rats." *Biological trace element research*, 160(2): 250-7. doi:10.1007/s12011-014-0040-6.

Dewey, W. A. 1997. *Practical Homeopathic Therapeutics*, Student Economic. B. Jain.

Diaz, Kristina. n.d. "Smoking and Sleep." American Sleep Association. Accessed Sept. 28, 2022. https://www.sleepassociation.org/blog-post/smoking-and-sleep/.

Dick-Kronenberg, L. 2012. *The Ultimate Text in Constitutional Hydrotherapy: A 100-Year Old Tradition of Clinical Practice.* Carroll Institute of Natural Healing.

Dimidi, Eirini, et al. n.d. "Fermented Foods: Definitions and Characteristics, Impact on the Gut Microbiota and Effects on Gastrointestinal Health and Disease." *Nutrients*, 11(8): 1806. doi:10.3390/nu11081806.

Domínguez-López, Inés, et al. 2020. "Effects of Dietary Phytoestrogens on Hormones Throughout a Human Lifespan: A Review." *Nutrients*, 12(8): 2456. doi:10.3390/nu12082456.

Dording, Christina M., et al. 2008. "A Double-Blind, Randomized, Pilot Dose-Finding Study of Maca Root (L. Meyenii) for the Management of SSRI-Induced Sexual Dysfunction." *CNS Neuroscience and Therapeutics*, 14(3): 182-91. doi:10.1111/j.1755-5949.2008.00052.x.

Dyall, Simon C. 2015. "Long-Chain Omega-3 Fatty Acids and The Brain: A Review of the Independent and Shared Effects of EPA, DPA and DHA." *Frontiers in Aging Neuroscience*, 7(52). doi:10.3389/fnagi.2015.00052.

Editors of Encyclopedia Britannica. 2022. "Clover Plant". *Britannica*. https://www.britannica.com/plant/clover-plant#ref89879.

Ekholm, P., H. Reinivuo, P. Mattila, H. Pakkala, J. Koponen, A. Happonen, J. Hellstrom, M. L. Ovaskainen. 2007. "Changes in the Mineral and Trace Element Contents of Cereals, Fruits and Vegetables in Finland." *Journal of Food Composition and Analysis*, Sept. 01, 2007, 20(6): 487-495.

Elliot, William J., et al. 2004. "Graded Blood Pressure Reduction in Hypertensive Outpatients Associated With Use of a Device to Assist With Slow Breathing." Greenwich, Conn.: *Journal of Clinical Hypertension*, 6(10): 553-61. doi:10.1111/j.1524-

6175.2004.03553.x.

Engels, Gail, et al. n.d. "Psyllium." Accessed Aug. 8, 2022. https://www.herbalgram.org/resources/herbalgram/issues/117/table-of-contents/hg117-herbprofile/.

Environmental Protection Agency. n.d. "Contaminated Lands." Last modified Sept. 28, 2021. https://www.epa.gov/report-environment/contaminated-land.

European Medicines Agency. 2014. "Assessment Report on Rubus Idaeus L., Folium." https://www.ema.europa.eu/en/documents/herbal-report/final-assessment-report-rubus-idaeus-l-folium_en.pdf.

Evered, David, Sara Harnett, and Ciba Foundation. 1988. *Cyanide Compounds in Biology*. J. Wiley. https://doi.org/10.1002/9780470513712.

Falk Symposium and K. W. Bock. 1991. *Hepatic Metabolism and Disposition of Endo- and Xenobiotics: Proceedings of the 57th Falk Symposium Held in Freiburg-Im-Breisgau Germany, October 8-10 1990*. Kluwer Academic.

Fernández, María Del Mar, et al. 2019. "Tobacco Consumption and Premenstrual Syndrome: A Case-Control Study." *PloS One*, 14(6): e0218794. doi:10.1371/journal.pone.0218794.

Ferreira, Mandy and Elizabeth Bennett. n.d. "Everything You Need to Know About the Oil Cleansing Method". *Healthline*. Reviewed Jan. 28, 2022. https://www.healthline.com/health/oil-cleansing-method#how-to-use.

Fiorini, Ana C., et al. 2016. "Can You Hear Me Now? The Quest for Better Guidance on Omega-3 Fatty Acid Consumption to Combat Hearing Loss." *Clinics (São Paulo, Brazil)*, 71(8): 420-2. doi:10.6061/clinics/2016(08)01.

Fleming, Althea, ND. 2018. *Advanced Topics in Geriatric Medicine Notes*.

Foulkes, E. C. 1990. *Biological Effects of Heavy Metals*. CRC Press.

Fowdar, Kaushal, et al. 2017. "The Effect of N-Acetylcysteine on Exacerbations of Chronic Obstructive Pulmonary Disease: A Meta-Analysis and Systematic Review." *Heart and Lung: The Journal Of Critical Care*, 46(2): 120-128. doi:10.1016/j.hrtlng.2016.12.004.

Fowles, J., and E. Dybing. 2003. "Application of Toxicological Risk Assessment Principles to the Chemical Constituents of Cigarette Smoke." *Tobacco Control* 12(4): 424-30. doi:10.1136/tc.12.4.424.

Fu, Zhenna, et al. 2018. "Effects of Total Flavonoids of Raspberry on Perimenopausal Model in Mice." *Saudi Journal of Biological Sciences*, 25(3): 487-492. doi:10.1016/j.sjbs.2017.08.009.

Furlanetto, K. C., L. C. Mantoani, G. Bisca, A. A. Morita, J. Zabatiero, M. Proença, ... F. Pitta. 2014. "Reduction of Physical Activity in Daily Life and Its Determinants in Smokers Without Airflow Obstruction." *Respirology, 19(3): 369–375*. doi:10.1111/resp.12236.

Gaby, A. 2017. *Nutritional Medicine*, 2nd ed. Fritz Perlberg Publishing.

Galzigna, L., C. Ceschi-Berrini, E. Moschin, and C. Tolomio. 1998. "Thermal Mud-Pack as an Anti-Inflammatory Treatment". *Biomedicine and Pharmacotherapy, 52(9): 408–409*. doi:10.1016/s0753-3322(99)80010-9.

Geller, Stacie E., et al. 2009. "Safety and Efficacy of Black Cohosh and Red Clover for the Management of Vasomotor Symptoms: A Randomized Controlled Trial." New York: *Menopause*, 16(6): 1156-66. doi:10.1097/gme.0b013e3181ace49b.

Giacosa, A., and M. Rondanelli. 2010. "The Right Fiber for the Right Disease". *Journal of Clinical Gastroenterology*, 44: S58–S60. doi:10.1097/mcg.0b013e3181e123e7.

Gill, S. K., M. Rossi, B. Bajka, and K. Whelan. 2020. "Dietary Fibre in Gastrointestinal Health and Disease". *Nature Reviews Gastroenterology and Hepatology*. doi:10.1038/s41575-020-00375-4.

Glennon, Sarah-Grace, et al. 2019. "Chronic Cigarette Smoking Associates Directly and Indirectly with Self-Reported Olfactory Alterations: Analysis of the 2011-2014 National Health and Nutrition Examination Survey." *Nicotine and Tobacco Research: Official Journal of the Society for Research on Nicotine and Tobacco*, 21(6): 818-827. doi:10.1093/ntr/ntx242.

Gohil, Kashmira J., et al. 2010. "Pharmacological Review on Centella Asiatica: A Potential Herbal Cure-All." *Indian Journal of Pharmaceutical Sciences*, 72(5): 546-56. doi:10.4103/0250-474X.78519.

Gomes, Celso de Sousa Figueiredo. 2018. "Healing and Edible Clays: A Review of Basic Concepts, Benefits and Risks." *Environmental Geochemistry and Health*, 40(5): 1739-1765. doi:10.1007/s10653-016-9903-4.

Gonzales, Gustavo F. 2012. "Ethnobiology and Ethnopharmacology of Lepidium Meyenii (Maca), a Plant From the Peruvian Highlands." *Evidence-Based Complementary and Alternative Medicine: eCAM*, 2012: 193496. doi:10.1155/2012/193496.

Grabhorn, L. 2005. *Excuse Me Your Life is Waiting: The Astonishing Power of Positive Feelings*. Hodder Mobius.

Gray, J. C., M. Thompson, C. Bachman, et al. 2020. "Associations of Cigarette Smoking With Gray and White Matter in the Uk Biobank". *Neuropsychopharmacol*, 45: 1215–1222. https://doi.org/10.1038/s41386-020-0630-2.

Grillo, Calogero, et al. 2019. "Influence of Cigarette Smoking on Allergic Rhinitis: A Comparative Study on Smokers and Non-Smokers." *Acta Bio-Medica: Atenei Parmensis*, 90(7-S): 45-51. doi:10.23750/abm.v90i7-S.8658.

Gulec, M., H. Ozkol, Y. Selvi, Y. Tuluce, A. Aydin, L. Besiroglu, and P. G. Ozdemir. 2012. "Oxidative Stress in Patients with Primary Insomnia". *Progress in Neuro-Psychopharmacology and Biological Psychiatry*, 37(2): 247–251. https://doi.org/10.1016/j.pnpbp.2012.02.011.

Gunavante, S. M. 1999. *The "Genius" of Homoeopathic Remedies*, reprint. Jain.

Gupta, P., D. K. Yadav, K. B. Siripurapu, G. Palit, and R. Maurya. 2007. "Constituents of Ocimum Sanctum with Antistress Activity". *Journal of Natural Products*, 70(9): 1410–1416. doi:10.1021/np0700164.

Hahnemann, S. 1880. *Materia Medica Pura: In 2 Vols*. Gould.

Hahnemann, S. 1996. *Organon of the Medical Art*, edited and annotated by W. B. O'Reilly. California: Birdcage Books.

Hajdusianek, W., A. Żórawik, M. Waliszewska-Prosół, R. Poręba, and P. Gać. 2021. "Tobacco and Nervous System Development and Function-New Findings 2015-2020". *Brain Sciences*, 11(6): 797. https://doi.org/10.3390/brainsci11060797.

Haramaki, N., et al. 2001. "Long-Term Smoking Causes Nitroglycerin Resistance in Platelets by Depletion of Intraplatelet Glutathione." *Arteriosclerosis, Thrombosis, and Vascular Biology*, 21(11): 1852-6. doi:10.1161/hq1001.097021.

Harris, Kindred K., et al. 2016. "Metabolic Effects of Smoking Cessation." *Nature Reviews, Endocrinology*, 12(5): 299-308. doi:10.1038/nrendo.2016.32.

Harvard, T. H. Chan: School of Public Health. n.d. "Vitamin E." *The Nutrition Source*. Accessed Jan 14, 2021. https://www.hsph.harvard.edu/nutritionsource/vitamin-e/.

Hashiguchi, M., Y. Ohta, M. Shimizu, et al. 2015. "Meta-Analysis of the Efficacy and Safety of Ginkgo Biloba Extract for the Treatment of Dementia". *J Pharm Health Care Sci*, 1: 14. https://doi.org/10.1186/s40780-015-0014-7.

Hawkins J., C. Baker, L. Cherry and E. Dunne. 2018. "Black Elderberry (Sambucus Nigra) Supplementation Effectively Treats Upper Respiratory Symptoms: A Meta-Analysis of Randomized, Controlled Clinical Trials. *Complementary Therapies in Medicine*. https://doi.org/10.1016/j.ctim.2018.12.004.

Heartland Center for Reproductive Health. n.d. "How Does Magnesium Affect Female Fertility?" Reviewed Sept. 8, 2022. https://www.heartlandfertility.com/blog/2014/09/08/how-does-magnesium-affect-female-146078.

HeartMath. n.d. "The Science of HeartMath". Accessed Dec. 15, 2021. https://www.

heartmath.com/science/.

Helmenstine, Anne Marie, Ph.D. 2021. "The Chemical Composition of Air." *ThoughtCo*, Sep. 8, 2021. thoughtco.com/chemical-composition-of-air-604288.

Hemilä, H., J. Kaprio. 2008. "Vitamin E Supplementation and Pneumonia Risk in Males Who Initiated Smoking at an Early Age: Effect Modification by Body Weight and Dietary Vitamin C". *Nutr J*, 7(33). https://doi.org/10.1186/1475-2891-7-33.

Hemilä, Harri. 2020. "Vitamin E and Mortality in Male Smokers of the ATBC Study: Implications for Nutritional Recommendations." *Frontiers in Nutrition*, March 31, 2020, 7(36). doi:10.3389/fnut.2020.00036.

Hendricks G. 1995. *Conscious Breathing: Breathwork For Health Stress Release and Personal Mastery*. Bantam Books.

Hersey, P., D. Prendergast, and A. Edwards. 1983. "Effects of Cigarette Smoking on the Immune System: Follow-Up Studies in Normal Subjects After Cessation of Smoking". *Medical Journal of Australia*, 2(9): 425–429. https://doi.org/10.5694/j.1326-5377.1983.tb122565.x.

Heshmati, J., R. Omani-Samani, S. Vesali, S. Maroufizadeh, M. Rezaeinejad, M. Razavi, and M. Sepidarkish. 2018. "The Effects of Supplementation with Chromium on Insulin Resistance Indices in Women with Polycystic Ovarian Syndrome: A Systematic Review and Meta-Analysis of Randomized Clinical Trials". *Hormone and Metabolic Research*, 50(03): 193–200. doi:10.1055/s-0044-101835.

Hirode, G., Wong R.J. 2020. "Trends in the Prevalence of Metabolic Syndrome in the United States, 2011-2016". *JAMA*, 323(24): 2526–2528. doi:10.1001/jama.2020.4501.

Hoffmann, D. 1996. *The Complete Illustrated Holistic Herbal: A Safe and Practical Guide to Making and Using Herbal Remedies*. Element Books.

Hong, Heeok, et al. 2009. "Effects of Pumpkin Seed Oil and Saw Palmetto Oil in Korean Men With Symptomatic Benign Prostatic Hyperplasia." *Nutrition Research and Practice*, 3(4): 323-7. doi:10.4162/nrp.2009.3.4.323.

Houston, Mark. "The Role Of Magnesium in Hypertension and Cardiovascular Disease." Greenwich, Conn.: *Journal of Clinical Hypertension*, 13(11): 843-7. doi:10.1111/j.1751-7176.2011.00538.x.

https://www.webmd.com/smoking-cessation/ss/slideshow-ways-smoking-affects-looks. n.d. Reviewed Nov. 13, 2021. Accessed June 9, 2022.

Huang, Jiaqi, et al. 2019. "Relationship Between Serum Alpha-Tocopherol and Overall and Cause-Specific Mortality." *Circulation Research*, 125(1): 29-40. doi:10.1161/CIRCRESAHA.119.314944.

Huang, Zhenqiu, et al. 2022. "Single-Cell Analysis of Somatic Mutations in Human Bronchial Epithelial Cells in Relation to Aging and Smoking." *Nature Genetics*, April 11, 2022. DOI: 10.1038/s41588-022-01035-w.

Hudson, A. 2001-1994. *Lymphatic Drainage: Therapy i*. Triam Press.

Hulkkonen, S., J. Auvinen, J. Miettunen, et al. 2019. "Smoking is Associated with Ulnar Nerve Entrapment: A Birth Cohort Study". *Sci Rep*, 9: 9450. https://doi.org/10.1038/s41598-019-45675-1.

Hummel, M., et al. 2007. "Chromium in Metabolic and Cardiovascular Disease." *Hormone and Metabolic Research = Hormon- und Stoffwechselforschung = Hormones et Metabolisme*, 39(10): 743-51. doi:10.1055/s-2007-985847.

Hussain, Joy, and Marc Cohen. 2018. "Clinical Effects of Regular Dry Sauna Bathing: A Systematic Review." *Evidence-Based Complementary and Alternative Medicine: eCAM*,

2018: 1857413. doi:10.1155/2018/1857413.

Ianiro, Gianluca, et al. 2016. "Digestive Enzyme Supplementation in Gastrointestinal Diseases." *Current Drug Metabolism*, 17(2): 187-93. doi:10.2174/1389200217021601 14150137.

Iftikhar, Noreen. n.d. "Hyperthyroidism Diet." Reviewed March 10, 2021. https://www.healthline.com/health/hyperthyroidism-diet.

Integumentary System. n.d. Accessed May 27, 2022. https://courses.lumenlearning.com/wm-biology2/chapter/integumentary-system/.

International Foundation for Gastrointestinal Disorder. n.d. "IBS Facts and Statistics." Accessed Aug. 26, 2022. https://aboutibs.org/what-is-ibs/facts-about-ibs/.

IQWiG - Institute for Quality and Efficiency in Health Care. 2006. "How Does Our Sense of Taste Work? - NCBI Bookshelf". Bethesda: *National Library of Medicine*. Reviewed Aug 17, 2016. https://www.ncbi.nlm.nih.gov/books/NBK279408/.

Jalanka, Jonna, et al. 2019. "The Effect of Psyllium Husk on Intestinal Microbiota in Constipated Patients and Healthy Controls." *International Journal of Molecular Sciences*, 20(2): 433. doi:10.3390/ijms20020433.

Jalili, Cyrus, et al. 2014. "Protective Effect of Urtica Dioica L Against Nicotine-Induced Damage on Sperm Parameters, Testosterone and Testis Tissue in Mice." *Iranian Journal of Reproductive Medicine*, 12(6): 401-8.

Jaramillo, Joshua D., et al. 2015. "Reduced Bone Density and Vertebral Fractures in Smokers. Men and COPD Patients at Increased Risk." *Annals of the American Thoracic Society*, 12(5): 648-56. doi:10.1513/AnnalsATS.201412-591OC.

Jarić, Snežana, et al. 2018. "Traditional Wound-Healing Plants Used in the Balkan Region (Southeast Europe)." *Journal of Ethnopharmacology*, 211: 311-328. doi:10.1016/j.jep.2017.09.018.

Jarrett, Christian. 2015. *Great Myths of the Brain*. Chichester, West Sussex, UK; Malden, MA, USA: Wiley Blackwell.

Jeddy, Nadeem, et al. 2018. "Comparison of the Efficacy of Herbal Mouth Rinse with Commercially Available Mouth Rinses: A Clinical Trial." *Journal of Oral and Maxillofacial Pathology: JOMFP*, 22(3): 332-334. doi:10.4103/jomfp.JOMFP_303_18.

Jones, D. P., et al. 1992. "Glutathione in foods listed in the National Cancer Institute's Health Habits and History Food Frequency Questionnaire." *Nutrition and Cancer*, 17(1): 57-75. doi:10.1080/01635589209514173.

Jones, N. and J. Blagih, F. Zani, et al. 2021. "Fructose Reprogrammes Glutamine-Dependent Oxidative Metabolism to Support LPS-induced inflammation". *Nat Commun*, 12: 1209. https://doi.org/10.1038/s41467-021-21461-4.

Kahrilas, P. J. and R. R. Gupta. 1990. "Mechanisms of Acid Reflux Associated with Cigarette Smoking." *Gut*, 31(1): 4-10. doi:10.1136/gut.31.1.4.

Kalani, Amir, et al. 2012. "Ashwagandha Root in the Treatment of Non-Classical Adrenal Hyperplasia." *BMJ Case Reports*, 2012: bcr2012006989. doi:10.1136/bcr-2012-006989.

Kapoor, D., and T. H. Jones. 2005. "Smoking and Hormones in Health and Endocrine Disorders". *European Journal of Endocrinology*, 152(4): 491–499. doi:10.1530/eje.1.01867.

Karren, K. J. 2010. *Mind*, 4th ed. Benjamin Cummings.

Kasouni, Athanasia I., et al. 2021. "The Unexplored Wound Healing Activity of *Urtica dioica* L. Extract: An In Vitro and In Vivo Study." *Molecules (Basel, Switzerland)*, 26(20): 6248. doi:10.3390/molecules26206248.

Kaume, Lydia, et al. 2014 "Antioxidant-Rich Berries Exert Modest Bone Protective Effects in Postmenopausal Smokers Without Improving Biomarkers of Bone Metabolism." *Journal of Functional Foods*, 9: 202-210.

Kazazis, Christos E., et al. 2014. "The Therapeutic Potential of Milk Thistle in Diabetes." *The Review of Diabetic Studies: RDS*, 11(2): 167-74. doi:10.1900/RDS.2014.11.167.

Kennedy, David O., et al. 2020. "Acute and Chronic Effects of Green Oat (*Avena Sativa*) Extract on Cognitive Function and Mood During a Laboratory Stressor in Healthy Adults: A Randomized, Double-Blind, Placebo-Controlled Study in Healthy Humans." *Nutrients*, 12(6): 1598. doi:10.3390/nu12061598.

Kent, J. T. 1981. *Lectures on Homoeopathic Philosophy*, 2nd print ed. North Atlantic Books.

Khaleghi, Sara, et al. 2017. "Tribulus Terrestris Extract Improves Human Sperm Parameters In Vitro." *Journal of Evidence-Based Complementary and Alternative Medicine*, 22(3): 407-412. doi:10.1177/2156587216668110.

Khanh Nguyen, Jean Sparks, Felix O. Omoruyi. 2016. "Investigation of the Cytotoxicity, Antioxidative and Immune-Modulatory Effects of Ligusticum Porteri (Osha) Root Extract on Human Peripheral Blood Lymphocytes". *Journal of Integrative Medicine*, 14(6): 465-472. ISSN 2095-4964. https://doi.org/10.1016/S2095-4964(16)60280-7. (https://www.sciencedirect.com/science/article/pii/S2095496416602807).

Kim, Ji Young, et al. 2012. "Beneficial Effects of Korean Red Ginseng on Lymphocyte DNA Damage, Antioxidant Enzyme Activity, and LDL Oxidation in Healthy Participants: A Randomized, Double-Blind, Placebo-Controlled Trial." *Nutrition Journal*, 11: 47. doi:10.1186/1475-2891-11-47.

Kim, Victor, and Shawn D. Aaron. 2018. "What is a COPD Exacerbation? Current Definitions, Pitfalls, Challenges and Opportunities For Improvement." *The European Respiratory Journal*, 52(5): 1801-261. doi:10.1183/13993003.01261-2018.

Kim, W. K., T. M. Herfel, C. S. Dunkley, P. Y. Hester, T. D. Crenshaw, and S. C. and Ricke. 2008. "The Effects of Alfalfa-Based Molt Diets on Skeletal Integrity of White Leghorns". *Poultry Science*, 87(11): 2178–2185. doi:10.3382/ps.2008-00034.

Kim, Young-Nam, et al. 2016. "The Effects of Exercise Training Aad Acute Exercise Duration on Plasma Folate and Vitamin B12." *Nutrition Research and Practice*, 10(2): 161-6. doi:10.4162/nrp.2016.10.2.161.

Kirkland, Anna E., et al. 2018. "The Role of Magnesium in Neurological Disorders." *Nutrients*, 10(6): 730. doi:10.3390/nu10060730.

Kirschner-Hermanns, Ruth, et al. 2019. "WS PRO 160 I 120 mg (A Combination of Sabal and Urtica Extract) in Patients With LUTS Related to BPH." *Therapeutic Advances in Urology*, 11: 1756287219879533. doi:10.1177/1756287219879533.

Knackstedt, Lori A.., et al. 2009. "The Role of Cystine-Glutamate Exchange in Nicotine Dependence in Rats and Humans." *Biological Psychiatry*, 65(10): 841-5. doi:10.1016/j.biopsych.2008.10.040.

Kobayashi, Hiromitsu, et al. 2018. "Forest Walking Affects Autonomic Nervous Activity: A Population-Based Study." *Frontiers in Public Health*, 6: 278. doi:10.3389/fpubh.2018.00278.

Kogure, Mana, et al. 2021. "Sodium/Potassium Ratio Change was Associated With Blood Pressure Change: Possibility of Population Approach For Sodium/Potassium Ratio Reduction in Health Checkup." *Hypertension Research: Official Journal of the Japanese Society of Hypertension*, 44(2): 225-231. doi:10.1038/s41440-020-00536-7.

Köhrle, J. F. Jakob, B. Contempré, J. E. Dumont. 2005. "Selenium, The Thyroid, and the Endocrine System". *Endocrine Reviews*, 26(7): 944–984. https://doi.org/10.1210/er.2001-0034.

Kong, Yee Wen, et al. 2016. "Sodium and Its Role in Cardiovascular Disease - The Debate Continues." *Frontiers in Endocrinology*, 7: 164. doi:10.3389/fendo.2016.00164.

Kopittke, P. M., R. C. Dalal, D. Finn, and N. W. Menzies. 2017. "Global Changes in Soil Stocks of Carbon, Nitrogen, Phosphorus, and Sulphur as Influenced by Long-term Agricultural Production." *Global Change Biology*, 23(6): 2509–2519. https://doi.org/10.1111/gcb.13513.

Kovac, J. R., et al. 2015. "Effects of Cigarette Smoking on Erectile Dysfunction." *Andrologia*, 47(10): 1087-92. doi:10.1111/and.12393.

Kralik, A., K. Eder, and M. Kirchgessner. 1996. "Influence of Zinc and Selenium Deficiency on Parameters Relating to Thyroid Hormone Metabolism". *Hormone and Metabolic Research, 28(05): 223–226.* doi:10.1055/s-2007-979169.

Kronenbuerger, Martin and Manfred Pilgramm. 2022. "Olfactory Training". State Pearls Publishing LLC. Bethesda: *National Library of Medicine*. Revised Jan. 2022. https://www.ncbi.nlm.nih.gov/books/NBK567741/.

Krzyżanowska-Kowalczyk, Justyna, et al. 2018. "Novel Phenolic Constituents of *Pulmonaria officinalis* L. LC-MS/MS Comparison of Spring and Autumn Metabolite Profiles." *Molecules (Basel, Switzerland)*, 23(9): 2277. doi:10.3390/molecules23092277.

Krzyżanowska-Kowalczyk, Justyna, et al. 2021. "*Pulmonaria Obscura* and *Pulmonaria Officinalis* Extracts as Mitigators of Peroxynitrite-Induced Oxidative Stress and Cyclooxygenase-2 Inhibitors-In Vitro and in Silico Studies." *Molecules (Basel, Switzerland),* 26(3): 631. doi:10.3390/molecules26030631.

Ladybird Johnson Wildflower Center. n.d. "Urtica Dioica." The University of Texas at Austin. Accessed Nov. 18, 2021. https://www.wildflower.org/plants/result.php?id_plant=URDI.

Langade, D., S. Kanchi, J. Salve, K. Debnath, and D. Ambegaokar. 2019. "Efficacy and Safety of Ashwagandha (Withania Somnifera) Root Extract in Insomnia and Anxiety: A Double-Blind, Randomized, Placebo-Controlled Study". *Cureus*, 11(9): e5797. https://doi.org/10.7759/cureus.5797.

Langton, A. K., E. Tsoureli-Nikita, H. Merrick, X. Zhao, C. Antoniou, A. Stratigos, R. Akhtar, B. Derby, M. J. Sherratt, R. E. Watson, and C. E. Griffiths. 2020. "The Systemic Influence of Chronic Smoking on Skin Structure and Mechanical Function. *J. Pathol.*, 251: 420-428. https://doi.org/10.1002/path.5476.

LaPier, Rosalyn R. 2017. "Why is Water Sacred to Native Americans?" Fall 2017. https://editions.lib.umn.edu/openrivers/article/why-is-water-sacred-to-native-americans/.

Leach, Matthew J., and Vivienne Moore. 2012. "Black Cohosh (Cimicifuga Spp.) for Menopausal Symptoms." *The Cochrane Database of Systematic Review*, 2012(9): CD007244. doi:10.1002/14651858.CD007244.pub2.

Lee, Myeong Soo, et al. 2016. "The Use of Maca (Lepidium Mmeyenii) to Improve Semen Quality: A Systematic Review." *Maturitas*, 92: 64-69. doi:10.1016/j.maturitas.2016.07.013.

Lee, Nam-Hun, et al. 2012. "Safety and Tolerability of Panax Ginseng Root Extract: A Randomized, Placebo-Controlled, Clinical Trial in Healthy Korean Volunteers." New York: *Journal of Alternative and Complementary Medicine*, 18(11): 1061-9. doi:10.1089/acm.2011.0591.

Leeuwendaal, N. K., C. Stanton, P. W. O'Toole, and T. P. Beresford. 2022. "Fermented Foods, Health and the Gut Microbiome". *Nutrients, 14*(7): 1527. https://doi.org/10.3390/nu14071527.

Leung, Angela M., et al. 2012. "History of U.S. Iodine Fortification and Supplementation." *Nutrients,* 4(11): 1740-6. doi:10.3390/nu4111740.

Leventhal, Adam M., and Michael J. Zvolensky. 2015. "Anxiety, Depression, and Cigarette Smoking: A Transdiagnostic Vulnerability Framework to Understanding Emotion-Smoking Comorbidity." *Psychological Bulletin*, 141(1): 176-212. doi:10.1037/bul0000003.

Li, Diandian, Dan Xu, Tao Wang, Yongchun Shen, Shujin Guo, Xue Zhang, Lingli Guo, Xiaoou Li, Lian Liu, Fuqiang Wen. 2014. Silymarin Attenuates Airway Inflammation Induced by Cigarette Smoke in Mice. *Inflammation*, 38(2), 871–878. doi:10.1007/s10753-014-9996-9.

Li, Jun, et al. 2009. "Effect of Dietary Selenium and Cigarette Smoke on Pulmonary Cell Proliferation in Mice." *Toxicological Sciences: An Official Journal of the Society of Toxicology*, 111(2): 247-53. doi:10.1093/toxsci/kfp151.

Li, Qing, et al. 2011. "Acute Effects Of Walking In Forest Environments On Cardiovascular and Metabolic Parameters." *European Journal Of Applied Physiology*, 111(11): 2845-53. doi:10.1007/s00421-011-1918-z.

Li, Xiaowen, et al. 2020. "Association Between Smoking and Noise-Induced Hearing Loss: A Meta-Analysis of Observational Studies." *International Journal of Environmental Research and Public Health*, 17(4): 1201. doi:10.3390/ijerph17041201.

Lin, Tzu-Kai, et al. 2017. "Anti-Inflammatory and Skin Barrier Repair Effects of Topical Application of Some Plant Oils." *International Journal of Molecular Sciences*, 19(1): 70. doi:10.3390/ijms19010070.

Lin, You-Shuei, et al. 2021. "Coenzyme Q_{10} Amends Testicular Function and Spermatogenesis in Male Mice Exposed to cigarette Smoke by Modulating Oxidative Stress and Inflammation." *American Journal of Translational Research*, 13(9): 10142-10154.

Lindlahr, H. and J. C. P. Proby. 1993. *Philosophy of Natural Therapeutics*. C.W. Daniel.

Lindlahr, H. and V. H. Lindlahr. 1931. *The Practice of Nature Cure*, revised and edited by Victor H. Lindlahr, 27th ed. Nature Cure Library.

Link, Rachael. 2018. "8 Health Benefits of Fasting, Backed by Science." *Healthline*, May 30, 2018. https://www.healthline.com/nutrition/fasting-benefits#TOC_TITLE_HDR_6.

Link, Rachel, et al. n.d. "Adrenal Fatigue Diet". Reviewed Oct. 1, 2021. https://www.healthline.com/health/adrenal-fatigue-diet#foods-to-eat.

Linus Pauling Institute: Oregon State University. 2022. "Vitamin E and Skin Health". Feb. 16, 2022. https://lpi.oregonstate.edu/mic/health-disease/skin-health/vitamin-E.

Linus Pauling Institute: Oregon State University. n.d. "Vitamin E". Reviewed May 2015. https://lpi.oregonstate.edu/mic/vitamins/vitamin-E.

Lipa, Katarzyna, et al. 2021. "Does Smoking Affect Your Skin?." *Postępy Dermatologii I Alergologii*, 38(3): 371-376. doi:10.5114/ada.2021.103000.

Lipa, Katarzyna, N. Zając W. Owczarek, P. Ciechanowicz, E. Szymanska, I. Walecka. 2021. "Does Smoking Affect Your Skin?". *Postępy Dermatologii I Alergologii*, 38(3): 371-376. doi:10.5114/ada.2021.103000.

Liu, Meixi, et al. 2019. "Magnesium and Liver Disease." *Annals of Translational Medicine*, 7(20): 578. doi:10.21037/atm.2019.09.70.

Lockett, Eleesha. n.d. "Grounding: Exploring Earthing Science and the Benefits Behind It". *Healthline*. Reviewed Aug. 30, 2019. https://www.healthline.com/health/grounding#benefits.

Lopresti, A. L., S. J. Smith, and P. D. Drummond. 2021. "Modulation of the Hypothalamic–Pituitary–Adrenal (HPA) Axis by Plants and Phytonutrients: A Systematic Review of Human Trials. *Nutritional Neuroscience*. 1-27. doi:10.1080/1028415x.2021.1892253.

Luo, Jing, et al. 2021. "Dietary Anti-Aging Polyphenols and Potential Mechanisms." *Antioxidants (Basel, Switzerland)*, 10(2): 283. doi:10.3390/antiox10020283.

Luper, S. 1998. "A Review of Plants Used in the Treatment of Liver Disease: Part 1." *Alternative Medicine Review: A Journal of Clinical Therapeutic*, 3(6): 410-21.

Lushchak, Volodymyr I. 2012. "Glutathione Homeostasis and Functions: Potential Targets for Medical Interventions." *Journal of Amino Acids,* 2012: 736837. doi:10.1155/2012/736837.

Lv, Junwei, et al. 2018. "Pharmacological Review on Asiatic Acid and Its Derivatives: A Potential Compound." *SLAS Technology,* 23(2): 111-127. doi:10.1177/2472630317751840.

Ma, Xiao, et al. 2017. "The Effect of Diaphragmatic Breathing on Attention, Negative Affect and Stress in Healthy Adults." *Frontiers in Psychology,* 8: 874. doi:10.3389/fpsyg.2017.

Mahmood, Khalid, et al. n.d. "Association of Cigarette Smoking with Irritable Bowel Syndrome: A Cross-Sectional Study." *Medical Journal of the Islamic Republic of Iran,* 34: 72. doi:10.34171/mjiri.34.72.

Mancini, Edele, et al. 2017. "Green Tea Effects on Cognition, Mood and Human Brain Function: A Systematic Review." *Phytomedicine: International Journal of Phytotherapy and Phytopharmacology,* 34: 26-37. doi:10.1016/j.phymed.2017.07.008

Mardikar, B. R. and University of Poona. 1989. *Krishna Tulas (Ocimum Sanctum) a Monograph.* Interdisciplinary School of Ayurvedic Medicine University of Poona.

Martin J., Wang Z. Q., X. H. Zhang, et al. 2006. "Chromium Picolinate Supplementation Attenuates Weight Gain and Increases Insulin Sensitivity in Subjects With Type 2 Diabetes". *Diabetes Care,* 29(8):1826-1832.

Marz R. B. 1999. *Medical Nutrition From Marz: A Textbook in Clinical Nutrition,* 2nd ed. Omni-Press.

May, James M., and Fiona E. Harrison. 2013. "Role of Vitamin C in the Function of the Vascular Endothelium." *Antioxidants and Redox Signaling,* 19(17): 2068-83. doi:10.1089/ars.2013.5205.

Mayo Clinic. 2008. "Enhance Healing Through Guided Imagery." *ScienceDaily,* Jan. 7, 2008. www.sciencedaily.com/releases/2008/01/080104123246.htm.

Mayo Clinic. n.d. "Coenzyme Q10." Accessed Jan. 27, 2022. https://www.mayoclinic.org/drugs-supplements-coenzyme-q10/art-20362602.

McClure, J. B., G. Divine, G. Alexander, D. Tolsma, S. J. Rolnick, M. Stopponi, ... C. Johnson. 2009. A Comparison of Smokers' and Nonsmokers' Fruit and Vegetable Intake and Relevant Psychosocial Factors. *Behavioral Medicine,* 35(1): 14–22. doi:10.3200/bmed.35.1.14-22.

McDaniel, J. C., and K. K. Browning. 2014. Smoking, Chronic Wound Healing, and Implications for Evidence-Based Practice. *Journal of Wound, Ostomy, and Continence Nursing: Official Publication of The Wound, Ostomy and Continence Nurses Society,* 41(5): 415–E2. https://doi.org/10.1097/WON.0000000000000057.

McGlory, Chris, et al. 2019. "The Influence of Omega-3 Fatty Acids on Skeletal Muscle Protein Turnover in Health, Disuse, and Disease." *Frontiers in Nutrition,* 6: 144. doi:10.3389/fnut.2019.00144.

Medline Plus. n.d. "Vitamin C." Revised March 11, 2021. https://medlineplus.gov/ency/article/002404.htm.

Mendes, Liliane Ps., et al. 2019. "Effects of Diaphragmatic Breathing With and Without Pursed-Lips Breathing in Subjects With COPD." *Respiratory Care,* 64(2): 136-144. doi:10.4187/respcare.06319.

Mills, S. and K. Bone. 2000. *Principles and Practice of Phytotherapy: Modern Herbal Medicine.* Churchill Livingstone.

Mills S. 1991. *Out Of The Earth: The Essential Book of Herbal Medicine.* Viking Arkana Penguin.

Mills S. and Bone K. 2000. *Principles and Practice of Phytotherapy: Modern Herbal Medicine*. Churchill Livingstone.

Miranda, Cristobal L., et al. 2009. "Ascorbic Acid Promotes Detoxification and Elimination of 4-Hydroxy-2(E)-Nonenal in Human Monocytic THP-1 Cells." *Chemical Research in Toxicology*, 22(5): 863-74. doi:10.1021/tx900042u.

Mokhtari, V., Afsharian, P., Shahhoseini, M., Kalantar, S. M., and Moini, A. 2017. "A Review on Various Uses of N-Acetyl Cysteine". *Cell journal*, 19(1): 11–17. https://doi.org/10.22074/cellj.2016.4872.

Monograph. "Sambucus Nigra (Elderberry)". 2005. *Alternative Medicine Review: A Journal of Clinical Therapeutic*, 10(1): 51–54.

Moolla, A., and A. M. Viljoen. 2008. "'Buchu' – Agathosma Betulina and Agathosma Crenulata (Rutaceae): A Review." *Journal of Ethnopharmacology*, 119(3), 413–419. doi:10.1016/j.jep.2008.07.036.

Moore, M. 1997. *Specific Indications for Herbs in General Use*. Bisbee, ARI, USA: Southwest School of Botanical Medicine.

Moosavi, Maryam. 2017. "Bentonite Clay as a Natural Remedy: A Brief Review." *Iranian Journal of Public Health*, 46(9): 1176-1183.

Morris, P. E., and Bernard, G. R. 1994. "Significance of Glutathione in Lung Disease and Implications for Therapy". *The American Journal of the Medical Sciences*, 307(2): 119–127. https://doi.org/10.1097/00000441-199402000-00010.

Mostafa, T., et al. 2006. "Effect of Smoking on Seminal Plasma Ascorbic Acid in Infertile and Fertile Males." *Andrologia*, 38(6): 221-4. doi:10.1111/j.1439-0272.2006.00744.x.

Mullin, James M., et al. 2016. "Methionine Restriction Fundamentally Supports Health by Tightening Epithelial Barriers." *Annals of the New York Academy of Sciences*, 1363: 59-67. doi:10.1111/nyas.12955.

Murray M. T., Pizzorno J. E., and Pizzorno L. 2005. *The Encyclopedia of Healing Foods*. Atria Books.

Murray M. T. 1997. *Chronic Candidiasis: Your Natural Guide to Healing With Diet Vitamins Minerals Herbs Exercise and Other Natural Methods*. Prima Health.

Myers, Jonathan, et al. 2019. "Physical Activity, Cardiorespiratory Fitness, and the Metabolic Syndrome." *Nutrients*, 11(7): 1652. doi:10.3390/nu11071652.

Myung, Seung-Kwon, et al. 2021. "Calcium Supplements and Risk of Cardiovascular Disease: A Meta-Analysis of Clinical Trials." *Nutrients*, 13(2): 368. doi:10.3390/nu13020368.

Naik, P. and L. Cucullo. "Pathobiology of Tobacco Smoking and Neurovascular Disorders: United Strings and Alternative Products". *Fluids Barriers CNS*, 12(25). https://doi.org/10.1186/s12987-015-0022-x.

Naiz, A., et al. 2012. "Anthelmintic and Relaxant Activities of *Verbascum Thapsus* Mullein." *BMC Complement Altern Med.*, March 30, 2012. doi: 10.1186/1472-6882-12-29.

Naomi, Ruth, et al. 2021. "Probiotics for Alzheimer's Disease: A Systematic Review." *Nutrients*, 14(1): 20. doi:10.3390/nu14010020.

Narkiewicz, K., P. J. H. Van De Borne, M. Hausberg, R. L. Cooley, M. D. Winniford, D. E. Davison, and V. K. Somers. 1998. "Cigarette Smoking Increases Sympathetic Outflow in Humans". *Circulation*, 98(6): 528–534. https://doi.org/10.1161/01.CIR.98.6.528.

National Center for Chronic Disease Prevention and Health Promotion (US) Office on Smoking and Health. 2014. "The Health Consequences of Smoking—50 Years of Progress: A Report of the Surgeon General." *Atlanta (GA): Centers for Disease Control and Prevention* (US). https://www.ncbi.nlm.nih.gov/books/NBK179276/.

National Center for Complementary and Integrative Health. n.d. "Black Cohosh." Reviewed May 2020. https://www.nccih.nih.gov/health/black-cohosh.

National Center for Complementary and Integrative Medicine. n.d. "Chasteberry." Reviewed July 2022. https://www.nccih.nih.gov/health/chasteberry.

National Heart, Lung, and Blood Institute. n.d. "COPD". Accessed Oct. 13, 2021. https://www.nhlbi.nih.gov/health-topics/copd.

National Heart, Lung, and Blood Institute. n.d. "Metabolic Syndrome." Accessed Aug. 8, 2022. https://www.nhlbi.nih.gov/health/metabolic-syndrome.

National Institute of Diabetes and Digestive and Kidney Diseases. n.d. "Your Digestive System and How it Works." https://www.niddk.nih.gov/health-information/digestive-diseases/digestive-system-how-it-works.

National Institute of Health News in Health. n.d. "Making a Healthier Home: Cast Toxins From Your Living Space." Revised Dec. 2020. https://newsinhealth.nih.gov/2016/12/making-healthier-home.

National Institute of Health - Office of Dietary Supplements. n.d. "Chromium." Reviewed June 9, 2022. https://ods.od.nih.gov/factsheets/Chromium-HealthProfessional/.

National Institutes of Health. n.d. "Zinc: Fact Sheet for Professionals". Reviewed Dec. 7, 2021. https://ods.od.nih.gov/factsheets/Zinc-HealthProfessional/.

NATO Advanced Study Institute on Molecular Aspects of Monooxygenases and Bioactivation of Toxic Compounds Arınç Emel Schenkman J. B. Hodgson E. and North Atlantic Treaty Organization. 1991. *Molecular Aspects of Monooxygenases and Bioactivation of Toxic Compounds.* Plenum Press.

Nelson, T. M., et al. 2018. "Cigarette Smoking is Associated With an Altered Vaginal Tract Metabolomic Profile." *Scientific Reports,* Jan. 16, 2018, 8(1): 852. doi:10.1038/s41598-017-14943-3.

Nguyen, K., J. Sparks, and F. Omoruyi. 2017. "Effects of *Ligusticum Porteri* (Osha) Root Extract on Human Promyelocytic Leukemia Cells". *Pharmacognosy Research,* 9(2): 156–160. https://doi.org/10.4103/0974-8490.204641.

Nicols, Hannah. n.d. "How does yoga work?". Reviewed April 14, 2021. https://www.medicalnewstoday.com/articles/286745.

Nikkhah Bodagh, Mehrnaz, et al. 2018. "Ginger in Gastrointestinal Disorders: A Systematic Review of Clinical Trials." *Food Science and Nutrition,* 7(1): 96-108. doi:10.1002/fsn3.807.

Nogueira, Leonardo, et al. 2018. "Cigarette Smoke Directly Impairs Skeletal Muscle Function Through Capillary Regression and Altered Myofibre Calcium Kinetics in Mice." *The Journal of Physiology,* 596(14): 2901-2916. doi:10.1113/JP275888.

Northrop-Clewes, C.A., and D. I. Thurnham. 2007. "Monitoring Micronutrients in Cigarette Smokers". *Clinica Chimica Acta; International Journal of Clinical Chemistry,* 377: 1-2, 14-38.

Nystoriak, Matthew A., and Aruni Bhatnagar. 2018. "Cardiovascular Effects and Benefits of Exercise." *Frontiers in Cardiovascular Medicine,* 5: 135. doi:10.3389/fcvm.2018.00135.

Ody, P. 1993. *The Complete Medicinal Herbal.* DK Publishing.

Ömeroğlu Şimşek, Gökçen, et al. 2021. "Effects of Oral pH Changes on Smoking Desire." *Balkan medical journal,* 38(3): 165-170. doi:10.5152/balkanmedj.2021.20125.

Oranchuk, D. J., A. G. Storey, A. R. Nelson, and J. B. Cronin. 2018. "Isometric Training and Long-Term Adaptations; Effects of Muscle Length, Intensity and Intent: A Systematic Review". *Scandinavian Journal of Medicine and Science in Sports.* doi:10.1111/sms.13375.

Oregon State University: Linus Pauling Institute's Micronutrient Information Center. n.d. "Essential Fatty Acids." Accessed Jan. 26, 2022. https://lpi.oregonstate.edu/mic/other-nutrients/essential-fatty-acids.

Osborn, Corrine. n.d. "Eye Exercises: How-to, Efficacy, Eye Health, and More." Reviewed Sept. 29, 2018. https://www.healthline.com/health/eye-health/eyeexercises#exercises.

Oschman, James L., et al. 2015. "The Effects of Grounding (Earthing) on Inflammation, the Immune Response, Wound Healing, and Prevention and Treatment of Chronic Inflammatory and Autoimmune Diseases." *Journal of Inflammation Research,* 8: 83-96.

doi:10.2147/JIR.S69656.
Ozkol, Halil, et al. 2012. "Subacute Effect of Cigarette Smoke Exposure in Rats: Protection by Pot Marigold (Calendula Officinalis L.) Extract." *Toxicology and Industrial Health*, 28(1): 3-9. doi:10.1177/0748233711401263.
Packer L. and Colman C. 1999. *The Antioxidant Miracle: Your Complete Plan for Total Health and Healing*. Wiley.
Pal, S., and S. Radavelli-Bagatini. 2012. "Effects of Psyllium on Metabolic Syndrome Risk Factors". *Obesity Reviews*, 13(11): 1034–1047. doi:10.1111/j.1467-789x.2012.01020.x.
Panahi, Y., P. Kianpour, R. Mohtashami, S. L. Atkin, A. E. Butler, R. Jafari, R. Badeli, and A. Sahebkar. 2018. "Efficacy of Artichoke Leaf Extract in Non-Alcoholic Fatty Liver Disease: A Pilot Double-Blind Randomized Controlled Trial". *Phytotherapy Research*, 32(7): 1382–1387. doi:10.1002/ptr.6073.
Pani, Arianna, et al. 2020. "Inositol and Non-Alcoholic Fatty Liver Disease: A Systematic Review on Deficiencies and Supplementation." *Nutrients*, 12(11): 3379. doi:10.3390/nu12113379.
Parham, P. 2000. *The Immune System*. Garland Publishing: Current Trends.
Park, Hye Jung, et al. 2016. "Dietary vitamin C intake protects against COPD: the Korea National Health and Nutrition Examination Survey in 2012." *International Journal of Chronic Obstructive Pulmonary Disease*, 11: 2721-2728. doi:10.2147/COPD.S119448.
Park, Hyun Jun, et al. 2016. "Effects of Korean Red Ginseng on Semen Parameters in Male Infertility Patients: A Randomized, Placebo-Controlled, Double-Blind Clinical Study." *Chinese Journal of Integrative Medicine*, 22(7): 490-5. doi:10.1007/s11655-015-2139-9.
Park, Jae-Woo, et al. 2010. "Effects of Korean Red Ginseng on Dry Mouth: A Randomized, Double-Blind, Placebo-Controlled Trial." *Journal of Ginseng Research*, 34(3): 183–191. doi:10.5142/jgr.2010.34.3.183.
Park, Junhyung, et al. 2016. "The Effect of the Sodium to Potassium Ratio on Hypertension Prevalence: A Propensity Score Matching Approach." *Nutrients*, 8(8): 482. doi:10.3390/nu8080482.
Park, Kyungho. 2015. "Role of Micronutrients in Skin Health and Function." *Biomolecules and Therapeutics*, 23(3): 207-17. doi:10.4062/biomolther.2015.003.
Pegas, P. N., et al. 2012. "Could Houseplants Improve Indoor Air Quality In Schools?." *Journal Of Toxicology And Environmental Health, Part A*, 75(22-23): 1371-80. doi:10.1080/15287394.2012.721169.
Perkins, K. A. 1992. "Metabolic Effects of Cigarette Smoking." *Journal of Applied Physiology (Bethesda, Md.: 1985)*, 72(2): 401-9. doi:10.1152/jappl.1992.72.2.401.
Ph.D., K. M. 2020. *Nutrient-Depleted Soil: What it Means For Our Food*. Chris Kresser, Sept. 24, 2020. https://chriskresser.com/depletion-of-soil-and-what-can-be-done/.
Phares, D. L. 1868. "Ceanothus Americanus: Red Root, New Jersey Tea."*Atlanta Medical and Surgical Journal*, 9A(3): 129-131.
Phillips, Michael, Renee N. Cataneo, Beth Ann Ditkoff, Peter Fisher, Joel Greenberg, Ratnasiri Gunawardena, C. Stephan Kwon, Olaf Tietje, and Cynthia Wong. 2006. "Prediction of Breast Cancer Using Volatile Biomarkers in the Breath." *Breast Cancer Research and Treatment* 99, 1: 19–21. https://doi.org/10.1007/s10549-006-9176-1.
Phipps, W. R., et al. 1993. "Effect of flax Seed Ingestion on the Menstrual Cycle." *The Journal of Clinical Endocrinology and Metabolism*, 77(5): 1215-9. doi:10.1210/jcem.77.5.8077314.
Pittilo, Michael R. 2000. "Cigarette Smoking, Endothelial Injury and Cardiovascular Disease." *International Journal of Experimental Pathology*, 81(4): 219-30. doi:10.1046/j.1365-2613.2000.00162.x.
Pizzorno, J. E. and Murray M. T. 2013. *Textbook of Natural Medicine*, 4th ed. Elsevier/Churchill Livingstone.
Pizzorno, Joseph. 2014. "Glutathione!". Encinitas, Calif.: *Integrative Medicine*, 13(1): 8-12.

Pizzorno, Lara. 2015. "Nothing Boring About Boron." *Encintias: Integrative Medicine*, 14(4): 35-48.
Pizzorno J., M. Murray. 2013. *Glandular Therapy: Textbook of Natural Medicine*. St. Louis: Elsevier. 306-311.
Poensin, D., P. H. Carpentier, C. Féchoz, and S. Gasparini. 2003. "Effects of Mud Pack Treatment on Skin Microcirculation". *Joint Bone Spine*, 70(5): 367–370. doi:10.1016/s1297-319x(03)00064-2.
Polland, Carly. n.d. "Bioadaptive Medicine". Accessed June 30, 2022. https://bioadaptivemedicine.com/new-blog/thyroid-adrenal-connection.
Pomerleau, O. F. 1992. "Nicotine and the Central Nervous System: Biobehavioral Effects of Cigarette Smoking". *The American Journal of Medicine*, 93(1): S2–S7. https://doi.org/10.1016/0002-9343(92)90619-M.
Poorolajal, Jalal, and Nahid Darvishi. 2016. "Smoking and Suicide: A Meta-Analysis." *PloS One*, 11(7): e0156348. doi:10.1371/journal.pone.0156348.
Pothuraju, R., R. K. Sharma, J. Chagalamarri, S. Jangra, and P. Kumar Kavadi. 2013. "A Systematic Review Ofgymnema Sylvestre in Obesity and Diabetes Management". *Journal of the Science of Food and Agriculture*, 94(5): 834–840. doi:10.1002/jsfa.6458.
Powell, Alvin. 2022. "When Science Meets Mindfulness". *The Harvard Gazette*, April 4, 2022. https://news.harvard.edu/gazette/story/2018/04/harvard-researchers-study-how-mindfulness-may-change-the-brain-in-depressed-patients/.
Powell, Gregory L., et al. 2019. "Chronic Treatment With N-acetylcysteine Decreases Extinction Responding and Reduces Cue-Induced Nicotine-Seeking." *Physiological reports*, 7(1): e13958. doi:10.14814/phy2.13958.
Prasad, M. N. V. 2008. *Trace Elements as Contaminants and Nutrients: Consequences in Ecosystems and Human Health*. Wiley.
Prasad, Sahdeo, et al. 2014. "Recent Developments in Delivery, Bioavailability, Absorption and Metabolism of Curcumin: The Golden Pigment From Golden Spice." *Cancer Research and Treatment*, 46(1): 2-18. doi:10.4143/crt.2014.46.1.2.
Preedy, V. R. and R. R. Watson. 2010. *Handbook of Disease Burdens and Quality of Life Measures*. Springer.
Products, Center for Tobacco. 2021. "What It's Like to Quit Smoking." *FDA*, Aug. 2021. https://www.fda.gov/tobacco-products/health-effects-tobacco-use/what-its-quit-smoking.
Pullar, Juliet M., et al. 2017. "The Roles of Vitamin C in Skin Health." *Nutrients*, 9(8): 866. doi:10.3390/nu9080866.
Qayyum, Rahila., et al. 2016. "Mechanisms Underlying the Antihypertensive Properties of Urtica Dioica." *Journal of Translational Medicine*, 14(1): 254. doi:10.1186/s12967-016-1017-3.
Qiao, Z. D., J. B. Dai, and Z. X. Wang. 2015. "The Hazardous Effects of Tobacco Smoking on Male Fertility". *Asian Journal of Andrology*, 17(6), 954. doi:10.4103/1008-682x.150847.
Qiu, F., C. L. Liang, H. Liu, Y. Q. Zeng, S. Hou, S. Huang, X. Lai, and Z. Dai, Z. 2017. "Impacts of Cigarette Smoking on Immune Responsiveness: Up and Down or Upside Down?". *Oncotarget*, 8(1): 268–284. https://doi.org/10.18632/oncotarget.13613.
Rabinovitz, S. 2014. "Effects of Omega-3 Fatty Acids on Tobacco Craving in Cigarette Smokers: A Double-Blind, Randomized, Placebo-Controlled Pilot Study". *Journal of Psychopharmacology*, 28(8): 804–809. doi:10.1177/0269881114536477.
Raeeszadeh, Mahdieh, et al. 2022. "The Antioxidant Properties of Alfalfa (*Medicago Sativa* L.) and Its Biochemical, Antioxidant, Anti-Inflammatory, and Pathological Effects on Nicotine-Induced Oxidative Stress in the Rat Liver." *Oxidative Medicine and Cellular Longevity*, 2022: 2691577. doi:10.1155/2022/2691577.
Rahman, I., and MacNee, W. 1999. "Lung Glutathione and Oxidative Stress: Implications in Cigarette Smoke-Induced Airway Disease". *The American Journal of Physiology*, 277(6): L1067–L1088. https://doi.org/10.1152/ajplung.1999.277.6.L1067.

Rahman, I., and MacNee, W. 2000. "Oxidative Stress and Regulation of Glutathione in Lung Inflammation". *The European Respiratory Journal*, 16(3): 534–554. https://doi.org/10.1034/j.1399-3003.2000.016003534.x.

Raman, Ryan. n.d. "Best Diet for Hypothyroidism: Foods to Eat, Foods to Avoid." Reviewed June 17, 2021. https://www.healthline.com/nutrition/hypothyroidism-diet.

Rand, Allison L., and Penny A. Asbell. 2011. "Nutritional Supplements for Dry Eye Syndrome." *Current Opinion in Ophthalmology*, 22(4): 279-82. doi:10.1097/ICU.0b013e3283477d23.

Reed, S. 2009. *Essential Physiological Biochemistry: An Organ-Based Approach*. John Wiley and Sons. Accessed Aug. 29, 2022. http://www.myilibrary.com?id=230622&ref=toc.

Rezaei, Nima, and Amene Saghazadeh, eds. 2019. *Biophysics and Neurophysiology of the Sixth Sense*. Cham: Springer.

Robinson, V. S. 2011. *Natural Approaches to Healing Adrenal Fatigue*. Starflower.

Roche, L. 1998. *Meditation Made Easy*, 1st ed. San Francisco: Harper.

Rodick Tyler C., Donna R. Seibels, Jeganathan Ramesh Babu, Huggins Kevin W. Higgins, Guang Ren, and Suresh T. Mathews. 2018. "Potential Role of Coenzyme Q10 in Health and Disease Conditions. *Nutrition and Dietary Supplements*, 10:1-11 https://doi.org/10.2147/NDS.S112119.

Rodriguez-Fontan, F., B. Reeves, K. Tuaño, S. Colakoglu, L. D' Agostino, and R. Banegas. 2020. "Tobacco Use and Neurogenesis: A Theoretical Review of Pathophysiological Mechanism Affecting the Outcome of Peripheral Nerve Regeneration". *Journal of Orthopaedics*, 22: 59–63. doi:10.1016/j.jor.2020.03.026.

Rogers, John M. 2019. "Smoking and Pregnancy: Epigenetics and Developmental Origins of the Metabolic Syndrome." *Birth Defects Research*, 111(17): 1259-1269. doi:10.1002/bdr2.1550.

RX List. n.d. "Inositol." Accessed Aug. 9, 2022. https://www.rxlist.com/inositol/supplements.htm.

Sadeghi-Ardekani, K., M. Haghighi, and R. Zarrin. 2018. "Effects of Omega-3 Fatty Acid Supplementation on Cigarette Craving and Oxidative Stress Index in Heavy-Smoker Males: A Double-Blind, Randomized, Placebo-Controlled Clinical Trial". *Journal of Psychopharmacology*, 32(9): 995–1002. https://doi.org/10.1177/0269881118788806.

Saini, Rajiv. 2011. "Coenzyme Q10: The Essential Nutrient." *Journal of Pharmacy and Bioallied Sciences*, 3(3): 466-7. doi:10.4103/0975-7406.84471.

Sakhaei, Shahriar, et al. 2018. "The Impact of Pursed-lips Breathing Maneuver on Cardiac, Respiratory, and Oxygenation Parameters in COPD Patients." *Open Access Macedonian Journal of Medical Sciences*, 6: 1851-1856. doi:10.3889/oamjms.2018.407.

Saklayen M. G. 2018. The Global Epidemic of the Metabolic Syndrome. *Current hypertension reports*, 20(2): 12. https://doi.org/10.1007/s11906-018-0812-z.

Salem, M. B., H. Affes, K. Ksouda, R. Dhouibi, Z. Sahnoun, S. Hammami, and K. M. Zeghal. 2015. "Pharmacological Studies of Artichoke Leaf Extract and Their Health Benefits". *Plant Foods for Human Nutrition*, 70(4): 441–453. doi:10.1007/s11130-015-0503-8.

Salgado, R. M., et al. 2017 "Effect of Oral Administration of Tribulus Terrestris Extract on Semen Quality and Body Fat Index of Infertile Men." *Andrologia*, 49(5): 10.1111/and.12655. doi:10.1111/and.12655.

Saltman, P. D., and L. G. Strause. 1993. "The Role of Trace Minerals in Osteoporosis." *Journal of the American College of Nutrition*, 12(4): 384-9. doi:10.1080/07315724.1993.10718327.

Salve, Jaysing, et al. 2019. "Adaptogenic and Anxiolytic Effects of Ashwagandha Root Extract in Healthy Adults: A Double-Blind, Randomized, Placebo-Controlled Clinical Study." *Cureus*, 11(12): e6466. doi:10.7759/cureus.6466.

Sayette, Michael A., et al. 1019. "Pleasant Olfactory Cues Can Reduce Cigarette Craving." *Journal of Abnormal Psychology*, 128(4): 327-340. doi:10.1037/abn0000431.

Schectman, G., J. C. Byrd, and H. W. Gruchow. 1989. "The Influence of Smoking on Vitamin C Status in Adults". *American Journal of Public Health*, 79(2): 158–162. https://doi.org/10.2105/ajph.79.2.158.

Schmölz, Lisa, et al. 2016. "Complexity of Vitamin E Metabolism." *World Journal of Biological Chemistry*, 7(1): 14-43. doi:10.4331/wjbc.v7.i1.14.

Schroyens, F. 2007. *The Essential Synthesis*. Homeopathic Book.

Schuman-Olivier, Z.., L. E. Stoeckel, E. Weisz, and A. E. Evins. 2014. "Smoking Effects in the Human Nervous System". *The Effects of Drug Abuse on the Human Nervous System*. Elsevier: 333–365. https://doi.org/10.1016/B978-0-12-418679-8.00011-3

Schwalfenberg, Gerry K., and Stephen J. Genuis. 2017. "The Importance of Magnesium in Clinical Healthcare." *Scientifica* , 2017: 4179326. doi:10.1155/2017/4179326.

Schwartz, Mathieu, et al. 2020. "Interactions Between Odorants and Glutathione Transferases in the Human Olfactory Cleft". *Chemical Senses*, 45(8): 645–654. https://doi.org/10.1093/chemse/bjaa055.

Scoditti, Egeria, et al. 2019. "Role of Diet in Chronic Obstructive Pulmonary Disease Prevention and Treatment." *Nutrients*, 11(6): 1357. doi:10.3390/nu11061357.

Sears, Margaret E., et al. 2012. "Arsenic, Cadmium, Lead, and Mercury in Sweat: A Systematic Review." *Journal of Environmental and Public Health*, 2012: 184745. doi:10.1155/2012/184745.

Seddon, J. M., et al. 2001. "Dietary Fat and Risk for Advanced Age-Related Macular Degeneration." *Archives of Ophthalmology (Chicago, Ill.: 1960)*, 119(8): 1191-9. doi:10.1001/archopht.119.8.1191.

Seddon, Johanna M., et al. 2006. "Cigarette Smoking, Fish Consumption, Omega-3 Fatty Acid Intake, and Associations with Age-Related Macular Degeneration: The US Twin Study of Age-Related Macular Degeneration." *Archives of Ophthalmology (Chicago, Ill.: 1960)*, 124(7): 995-1001. doi:10.1001/archopht.124.7.995.

Shakeela Begum, Marthadu, Bulle Saradamma, Vaddi Damodara Reddy, Pannuru Padmavathi, Paramahamsa Maturu, Naresh babu Ellutla, Lokesh Thippannagari, N.C. Varadacharyulu. 2017. "Influence of Green Tea Consumption on Cigarette Smoking-Induced Biochemical Changes In Plasma And Blood". Clinical Nutrition Experimental, 16. 10.1016/j.yclnex.2017.10.002.

Shanb, Alsayed A., and Enas F Youssef. 2014. "The Impact of Adding Weight-Bearing Exercise Versus Nonweight Bearing Programs to the Medical Treatment of Elderly Patients with Osteoporosis." *Journal of Family and Community Medicine*, 21(3): 176-81. doi:10.4103/2230-8229.142972.

Shaw, Mary, et al. 2000. "Time for a Smoke? One Cigarette Reduces Your Life by 11 Minutes." *BMJ: British Medical Journal*, Jan. 2000, 320(7226): 53.

Shayganfard, M. 2021. "Are Essential Trace Elements Effective in Modulation of Mental Disorders? Update and Perspectives". *Biological Trace Element Research*. doi:10.1007/s12011-021-02733-y.

Shekoohi, Niloofar, et al. 2017. "Smoking Discriminately Changes the Serum Active and Non-Active Forms of Vitamin B12." *Acta Medica Iranica*, 55(6): 389-394.

Simopoulos, A. P. 2002. "The importance of the Ratio of Omega-6/Omega-3 Essential Fatty Acids." *Biomedicine and Pharmacotherapy = Biomedecine and Pharmacotherapie*, 56(8): 365-79. doi:10.1016/s0753-3322(02)00253-6.

Singh, P., B. Singh, R. Dave, and R. Udainiya. 2011. "The Impact of Yoga Upon Female Patients Suffering From Hypothyroidism". *Complementary Therapies in Clinical Practice*, 17(3): 132–134. doi:10.1016/j.ctcp.2010.11.004.

Singh, R., S. De, and A. Belkheir. 2013. "Avena Sativa (Oat), A Potential Neutraceutical and Therapeutic Agent: An Overview". *Critical Reviews in Food Science and Nutrition,*

53(2), 126-144. doi:10.1080/10408398.2010.526725.

Sinha, R., et al. 2018. "Oral Supplementation With Liposomal Glutathione Elevates Body Stores of Glutathione and Markers of Immune Function." *European Journal of Clinical Nutrition*, 72(1): 105-111. doi:10.1038/ejcn.2017.132.

Skosana, Bongekile, Yapo Aboua and Stefan Du Plessis. 2014." Buchu – The Multi-Purpose Ethnomedicinally Important Specie and Its Benefits in the Reproductive System". 10.5772/57233.

So, Seung-Ho, et al. 2018. "Red Ginseng Monograph." *Journal of Ginseng Research*, 42(4): 549-561. doi:10.1016/j.jgr.2018.05.002.

Sökeland, J. 2000. "Combined Sabal and Urtica Extract Compared With Finasteride in Men With Benign Prostatic Hyperplasia: Analysis of Prostate Volume and Therapeutic Outcome." *BJU International*, 86,(4): 439-42. doi:10.1046/j.1464-410x.2000.00776.x.

Solberg, Y., et al. 1998. "The Association Between Cigarette Smoking and Ocular Diseases." *Survey of Ophthalmology*, 42(6): 535-47. doi:10.1016/s0039-6257(98)00002-2.

Song, Chorong, et al. 2018. "Psychological Benefits of Walking Through Forest Areas." *International Journal of Environmental Research and Public Health*, 15(12): 2804. doi:10.3390/ijerph15122804.

Sonnenschmidt, R. 2009. *Liver and Gallbladder - Acquired Authority*, 1st English ed. Narayana.

Spitler, H. R. and American Naturopathic Association. 1948. *Basic Naturopathy; A Textbook*. American Naturopathic Assn.

Spravchikov, N., et al. 2001. "Glucose Effects on Skin Keratinocytes: Implications for Diabetes Skin Complications." *Diabetes*, 50(7): 1627-35. doi:10.2337/diabetes.50.7.1627.

Stämpfli, M. and G. Anderson. 2009. "How Cigarette Smoke Skews Immune Responses to Promote Infection, Lung Disease and Cancer". *Nat Rev Immunol*, 9: 377–384. https://doi.org/10.1038/nri2530.

Stechmiller, Joyce K., et al. 2005. "Arginine Supplementation and Wound Healing." *Nutrition in Clinical Practice: Official Publication of the American Society for Parenteral and Enteral Nutrition*, 20(1): 52-61. doi:10.1177/011542650502000152.

Stewart, P., R. Valentino, A. M. Wallace, D. Burt, C. L. Shackleton, and C. W. Edwards. 1987. "Mineralocorticoid Activity of Liquorice: 11-Beta-Hydroxysteroid Dehydrogenase Deficiency Comes of Age". *The Lancet, 330(8563): 821–824*. doi:10.1016/s0140-6736(87)91014-2.

Strum, S. B. 2021. "Serenoa Repens (Saw Palmetto) for Lower Urinary Tract Symptoms (LUTS): The Evidence for Efficacy and Safety of Lipidosterolic Extracts. Part II." *Uro*, 1(3):139-154. https://doi.org/10.3390/uro1030016.

Sun Boju, et al. 2020. "Therapeutic Potential of Centella Asiatica and Its Triterpenes: A Review". *Frontiers in Pharmacology*, 11. doi:10.3389/fphar.2020.568032.

Suzanne J. Einöther, Vanessa E. Martens. 2013. "Acute Effects of Tea Consumption on Attention and Mood". *The American Journal of Clinical Nutrition*, 98(6): 1700S–1708S. https://doi.org/10.3945/ajcn.113.058248.

Svartberg, Johan, and Rolf Jorde. 2007. "Endogenous Testosterone Levels and Smoking in Men. The Fifth Tromsø Study." *International Journal of Andrology*, 30(3): 137-43. doi:10.1111/j.1365-2605.2006.00720.x.

Sørensen L. T., U. B. Hemmingsen, L. T. Kirkeby, F. Kallehave, L. N. Jørgensen. 2005. "Smoking Is a Risk Factor for Incisional Hernia". *Arch Surg*, 140(2): 119–123.

doi:10.1001/archsurg.140.2.119.

Tabassum, Noor E., et al. 2022. "*Ginkgo Biloba*: A Treasure of Functional Phytochemicals with Multimedicinal Applications." *Evidence-Based Complementary and Alternative Medicine: eCAM*, 2022: 8288818. doi:10.1155/2022/8288818.

Talbot, Prue, and Karen Riveles. 2005. "Smoking and Reproduction: The Oviduct as a Target of Cigarette Smoke." *Reproductive Biology and Endocrinology*, 3. 52. Doi:10.1186/1477-7827-3-52.

Tang, Yi-Yuan, et al. 2009. "Central and Autonomic Nervous System Interaction is Altered by Short-Term Meditation." *Proceedings of the National Academy of Sciences of the United States of America*, 106(22): 8865-70. doi:10.1073/pnas.0904031106.

Tanvetyanon, Tawee, and Gerold Bepler. 2008. "Beta-Carotene in Multivitamins and the Possible Risk of Lung Cancer Among Smokers Versus Former Smokers: A Meta-Analysis and Evaluation of National Brands." *Cancer*, 113(1): 150-7. doi:10.1002/cncr.23527.

Tayade, Motilal. 2012. "Effect of Smoking on Nerve Conduction Velocity in Young Healthy Individuals". *International Journal of Current Research and Review*, 4: 57-61.

Taylor, Gemma, et al. 2014. "Change in Mental Health After Smoking Cessation: Systematic Review and Meta-Analysis." *BMJ (Clinical Research ed.)*, 348: g1151. doi:10.1136/bmj.g1151.

Tejapārakhījī, Saraśrī and Iyer K. 2008. *Complete Meditation: From Doing Meditation to Being Meditation*, 3rd ed. Wow Pub.

Tenório, Micaely Cristina Dos Santos, et al. 2021. "N-Acetylcysteine (NAC): Impacts on Human Health." *Antioxidants (Basel, Switzerland)*, 10(6): 967. doi:10.3390/antiox10060967.

The University of Sydney. n.d. Accessed Aug. 09, 2022. https://glycemicindex.com/about-gi/.

Thorup, Anne Cathrine, et al. 2015. "Intake of Novel Red Clover Supplementation for 12 Weeks Improves Bone Status in Healthy Menopausal Women." *Evidence-Based Complementary and Alternative Medicine: eCAM*, 2015: 689138. doi:10.1155/2015/689138.

Ticinesi, Andrea, et al. 2017. "Aging Gut Microbiota at the Cross-Road between Nutrition, Physical Frailty, and Sarcopenia: Is There a Gut-Muscle Axis?." *Nutrients*, 9(12): 1303. doi:10.3390/nu9121303.

Tiwari, Pragya, et al. 2014. "Phytochemical and Pharmacological Properties of Gymnema Sylvestre: An Important Medicinal Plant." *BioMed Research International*, 2014: 830285. doi:10.1155/2014/830285.

Tobacco. n.d. Accessed Sept. 2, 2021. https://www.who.int/news-room/fact-sheets/detail/tobacco.

Tomisawa, Toshiko, et al. 2019. "Effects of Blackcurrant Anthocyanin on Endothelial Function and Peripheral Temperature in Young Smokers." *Molecules (Basel, Switzerland)*, 24(23): 4295. doi:10.3390/molecules24234295.

Touvier, Mathilde, et al. 2005. "Dual Association of Beta-Carotene With Risk of Tobacco-Related Cancers in a Cohort of French Women." *Journal of the National Cancer Institute*, 97(18): 1338-44. doi:10.1093/jnci/dji276.

Trickey, Ruth. 2011. *Women, Hormones and the Menstrual Cycle*, 3rd ed. Trickey Enterprises; Victoria.

Trivedi, M. S., D. Holger, A. T. Bui, T. Craddock, and J. L. Tartar. 2017. "Short-Term Sleep

Deprivation Leads to Decreased Systemic Redox Metabolites and Altered Epigenetic Status. *PloS One*, *12*(7): e0181978. https://doi.org/10.1371/journal.pone.0181978.

Tungtrongchitr, R., P. Pongpaew, M. Soonthornruengyot, D. Viroonudomphol, N. Vudhivai, A. Tungtrongchitr, ... F. P. Schelp. 2003. "Relationship of Tobacco Smoking with Serum Vitamin B12, Folic Acid and Hematological Indices in Healthy Adults". *Public Health Nutrition*, 6(07). doi:10.1079/phn2003483.

Tyler, M. L. 2004. *Homeopathic Drug Picture*, 2004 ed. B. Jain.

Tziomalos, K. and F. Charsoulis. 2004. "Endocrine Effects of Tobacco Smoking". *Clinical Endocrinology*, 61: 664-674. https://doi.org/10.1111/j.1365-2265.2004.02161.x.

U.S. Department of Health and Human Services. 2010. *How Tobacco Smoke Causes Disease: The Biology and Behavioral Basis for Smoking-Attributable Disease: A Report of the Surgeon General*. Atlanta, GA: U.S. Department of Health and Human Services, Centers for Disease Control and Prevention, National Center for Chronic Disease Prevention and Health Promotion, Office on Smoking and Health.

U.S. Geological Survey. n.d. "The Water in You: Water and the Human Body." Accessed Nov. 25, 2021. https://www.usgs.gov/special-topic/water-science-school/science/water-you-water-and-human-body?qt-science_center_objects=0#qt-science_center_objects.

Ueha, Rumi, et al. 2020. "Effects of Cigarette Smoke on the Nasal Respiratory and Olfactory Mucosa in Allergic Rhinitis Mice." *Frontiers in neuroscience*, 14: 126. doi:10.3389/fnins.2020.00126.

United States Environmental Protection Agency. n.d. "Report on the Environment: Drinking Water." Last modified Sept. 28, 2021. https://www.epa.gov/report-environment/drinking-water.

Vanessa Garcia-Larsen, James F. Potts, et al. 2017. "Dietary antioxidants and 10-year lung function decline in adults from the ECRHS survey." *European Respiratory Journal*, 50(6): 1602286. DOI: 10.1183/13993003.02286-2016.

Vanvoorhis, B., J. Dawson, D. Stovall, A. Sparks, and C. Syrop. 1996. "The Effects Of Smoking on Ovarian Function and Fertility During Assisted Reproduction Cycles". *Obstetrics and Gynecology*, 88(5), 785–791. Doi:10.1016/0029-7844(96)00286-.

Van Wyk, B.-E. and Wink M. 2004. *Medicinal Plants of The World: An Illustrated Scientific Guide to Important Medicinal Plants and Their Uses*, 1st ed. Timber Press.

Vasey, C. 2009. *The Naturopathic Way: How to Detox Find Quality Nutrition and Restore Your Acid-Alkaline Balance*. Healing Arts Press.

Velussi, M., A. M. Cernigoi, L. Viezzoli, F. Dapas, C. Caffau, and M. Zilli. 1993. "Silymarin Reduces Hyperinsulinemia, Malondialdehyde Levels, and Daily Insulin Need in Cirrhotic Diabetic Patients". *Current Therapeutic Research*, 53(5): 533–545. doi:10.1016/s0011-393x(05)80660-5.

Venuprasad, M. P., H. K. Kandikattu, S. Razack, N. Amruta and F. Khanum. 2017. "Chemical Composition of Ocimum Sanctum by LC-ESI–MS/MS Analysis and Its Protective Effects Against Smoke Induced Lung And Neuronal Tissue Damage in Rats". *Biomedicine and Pharmacotherapy*, 91: 1–12. doi:10.1016/j.biopha.2017.04.011.

Wackerhage H. and M. J. Rennie. 2006. "How Nutrition and Exercise Maintain the Human Musculoskeletal Mass". *J Anat.*, 208(4): 451-458. doi:10.1111/j.1469-7580.2006.00544.x.

Wallace, Caroline J. K., and Roumen Milev. 2017. "The Effects of Probiotics on Depressive Symptoms in Humans: A Systematic Review." *Annals of General Psychiatry*, 16(14). doi:10.1186/s12991-017-0138-2.

Walter, Kimberly N., et al. 2012. "Elevated Thyroid Stimulating Hormone is Associated with Elevated Cortisol in Healthy Young Men and Women." *Thyroid Research*, 5(1): 13. doi:10.1186/1756-6614-5-13.

Wang, Jie, et al. 2013. "Effect of Crataegus Usage in Cardiovascular Disease Prevention:

An Evidence-Based Approach." *Evidence-Based Complementary and Alternative Medicine: eCAM,* 2013: 149363. doi:10.1155/2013/149363.

Wang, Pei-Wen, et al. 2019. "Red Raspberry Extract Protects the Skin against UVB-Induced Damage with Antioxidative and Anti-inflammatory Properties." *Oxidative Medicine and Cellular Longevity,* Jan 6, 2019. 9529676. doi:10.1155/2019/9529676.

Wathes, D. Claire, et al. 2007. "Polyunsaturated Fatty Acids in Male and Female Reproduction." *Biology of Reproduction,* 77(2): 190-201. doi:10.1095/biolreprod.107.060558.

Webb, G. P. 2006. *Dietary Supplements and Functional Foods.* Blackwell Pub.

Wells, Katie. 2014. "Deep Cleansing Mud Mask Ritual". *Wellness Mama,* Sept. 5, 2014. https://wellnessmama.com/beauty/mud-mask-recipe/.

Wendel, P. 1951. *Standardized Naturopathy.* Wendel.

Wetter, D. W. and T. B. Young. 1994. "The Relation Between Cigarette Smoking and Sleep Disturbance." *Preventive Medicine,* 23(3): 328-34. doi:10.1006/pmed.1994.1046.

Whitcroft K. L. and T. Hummel. 2020. "Olfactory Dysfunction in COVID-19: Diagnosis and Management." *JAMA.,* 323(24): 2512–2514. doi:10.1001/jama.2020.8391.

Wieland, L. S., V. Piechotta, T. Feinberg, E. Ludeman, B. Hutton, S. Kanji, D. Seely, and C. Garritty. 2021. "Elderberry for Prevention and Treatment of Viral Respiratory Illnesses: A Systematic Review". *BMC Complementary Medicine and Therapies, 21*(1): 112. https://doi.org/10.1186/s12906-021-03283-5.

Wilson, J. L. and Smart Publications. 2001. *Adrenal Fatigue: The 21st Century Stress Syndrome,* 1st ed. Smart Publications.

Wu, Wen-Huey, et al. 2006. "Sesame Ingestion Affects Sex Hormones, Antioxidant Status, and Blood Lipids in Postmenopausal Women." *The Journal of Nutrition,* 136(5): 1270-5. doi:10.1093/jn/136.5.1270.

Xu, Huan, et al. 2016. "Smoking Habits and Benign Prostatic Hyperplasia: A Systematic Review and Meta-Analysis of Observational Studies." *Medicine,* 95(32): e4565. doi:10.1097/MD.0000000000004565.

Xu, Yangying, et al. 2018. "Pretreatment With Coenzyme Q10 Improves Ovarian Response and Embryo Quality in Low-Prognosis Young Women With Decreased Ovarian Reserve: A Randomized Controlled Trial." *Reproductive Biology and Endocrinology: RB&E,* 16(1): 29. doi:10.1186/s12958-018-0343-0.

Yance, Donald. 2013. *Adaptogens in Medical Herbalism.* Rochester: Healing Arts Press. 438-444.

Yang, Hee Jung, et al. 2015. "Effects of Smoking on Menopausal Age: Results From the Korea National Health and Nutrition Examination Survey, 2007 to 2012." *Journal of Preventive Medicine and Public Health = Yebang Uihakhoe Chi,* 48(4): 216-24. doi:10.3961/jpmph.15.021.

Yanni Li, Yilun Chen, Dongxiao Sun-Waterhouse. 2022. "The Potential of Dandelion in the Fight Against Gastrointestinal Diseases: A Review". *Journal of Ethnopharmacology,* 293: 115272. ISSN 0378-8741. https://doi.org/10.1016/j.jep.2022.115272. https://pubmed.ncbi.nlm.nih.gov/35405251/.

Yazdanparast, Taraneh, et al. 2019. "Cigarettes Smoking and Skin: A Comparison Study of the Biophysical Properties of Skin in Smokers and Non-Smokers." *Tanaffos,* 18(2): 163-168.

Yin R. V., O. J. Phung. 2015. "Effect of Chromium Supplementation on Glycated Hemoglobin and Fasting Plasma Glucose in Patients With Diabetes Mellitus". *Nutrition Journal,* 14:14.

Zaccaro, Andrea, et al. 2018. "How Breath-Control Can Change Your Life: A Systematic Review on Psycho-Physiological Correlates of Slow Breathing." *Frontiers in Human Neuroscience,* 12: 353. doi:10.3389/fnhum.2018.00353.

Zamani, H., et al. 2021. "The Benefits and Risks of Beetroot Juice Consumption: A Systematic Review." *Critical Reviews in Food Science and Nutrition,* 61(5): 788-804. doi:10.1080/10408398.2020.1746629.

Zemmouri, Hanene, et al. 2017. "Urtica Dioica Attenuates Ovalbumin-Induced Inflammation and Lipid Peroxidation of Lung Tissues in Rat Asthma Model." *Pharmaceutical Biology,* 55(1): 1561-1568. doi:10.1080/13880209.2017.1310905.

Zenico, T., et al. 2009. "Subjective Effects of Lepidium Meyenii (Maca) Extract on Well-Being and Sexual Performances in Patients With Mild Erectile Dysfunction: A Randomised, Double-Blind Clinical Trial." *Andrologia* 41(2): 95-9. doi:10.1111/j.1439-0272.2008.00892.x.

Zhai, Qixiao, et al. 2015. "Dietary Strategies for the Treatment of Cadmium and Lead Toxicity." *Nutrients,* 7(1): 552-71. doi:10.3390/nu7010552.

Zhang, Xi, et al. 2016. "Effects of Magnesium Supplementation on Blood Pressure: A Meta-Analysis of Randomized Double-Blind Placebo-Controlled Trials." *Hypertension (Dallas, Tex. : 1979),* 68(2: 324-33. doi:10.1161/HYPERTENSIONAHA.116.07664.

Zhong, Shan, et al. 2015. "Effects of Schisandra Chinensis Extracts on Cough and Pulmonary Inflammation in a Cough Hypersensitivity Guinea Pig Model Induced by Cigarette Smoke Exposure." *Journal of Ethnopharmacology,* 165: 73-82. doi:10.1016/j.jep.2015.02.009.

Zhu, Lanlan, et al. 2021. "The Antioxidant N-Acetylcysteine Promotes Immune Response And Inhibits Epithelial-Mesenchymal Transition to Alleviate Pulmonary Fibrosis in Chronic Obstructive Pulmonary Disease By Suppressing The VWF/p38 MAPK Axis." *Molecular Medicine (Cambridge, Mass.),* 27(1): 97. doi:10.1186/s10020-021-00342-y.

Zita, C., Overvad, K., S. A. Mortensen, C. D. Sindberg, S. Moesgaard, and D. A. Hunter. 2003. "Serum Coenzyme Q10 Concentrations in Healthy Men Supplemented With 30 mg or 100 mg Coenzyme Q10 for Two Months in a Randomized Controlled Study". *BioFactors, 18(1-4):* 185–193. doi:10.1002/biof.5520180221.

Zubair, Ahmed Ratan, et al. 2021. Pharmacological Potential of Ginseng and Its Major Component Ginsenosides. *Journal of Ginseng Research,* 45(2): 199-210. https://doi.org/10.1016/j.jgr.2020.02.004.

Zuñiga, L. Y., M. González-Ortiz, and E. Martínez-Abundis. 2017. "Effect Of Gymnema Sylvestre Administration on Metabolic Syndrome, Insulin Sensitivity, and Insulin Secretion". *Journal of Medicinal Food,* 20(8): 750–754. doi:10.1089/jmf.2017.0001.

"Alfalfa." 2021. *MedlinePlus,* Sept. 24th, 2021. https://medlineplus.gov/druginfo/natural/19.html.

"Calorie." n.d. Merriam-Webster Dictionary, Accessed Aug. 1, 2022. https://www.merriam-webster.com/dictionary/calorie.

"Coenzyme q10". 2014. Linus Pauling Institute, April 28, 2014. https://lpi.oregonstate.edu/mic/dietary-factors/coenzyme-Q10.

"Colonic Enemas - A Naturopathic Treatment". 1998. *Townsend Letter for Doctors and Patients,* No. 180: 100-100.

"Flavonoids". n.d. Linus Pauling Institute. Oregon State University. Accessed Dec. 12, 2021. http://lpi.oregonstate.edu/infocenter/phytochemicals/flavonoids/.

"Global: Tobacco Market Value 2012-2025." n.d. *Statista.* Accessed Sept. 2, 2021. https://www.statista.com/forecasts/1098876/tobacco-global-market-value.

"How to Add More Fiber to Your Diet." n.d. Mayo Clinic. Accessed Aug. 20, 2022. https://www.mayoclinic.org/healthy-lifestyle/nutrition-and-healthy-eating/in-depth/fiber/art-20043983.

"Infrared Sauna Benefits vs Traditional Sauna Benefits – Which is Best?" n.d. Accessed Jan. 4, 2021. https://finnmarksauna.com/blogs/finnmark-blog/infrared-sauna-benefits-vs-traditional-sauna-benefits-which-is-best.

"Key Nutrients Necessary for Healthy Bones and Muscle." 2018. *London Osteoporosis Clinic,* May 3, 2018. https://www.londonosteoporosisclinic.com/key-nutritents-necessary-for-healthy-bones-and-muscle.

"Office of Dietary Supplements - Vitamin E." n.d. Accessed Jan. 7, 2022. https://ods.od.nih.gov/factsheets/VitaminE-HealthProfessional/.

"Peppermint." n.d. Accessed Aug. 26, 2022. https://www.britannica.com/plant/peppermint.

"Peppermint Oil." n.d. Accessed Aug. 26, 2022. https://www.nhs.uk/medicines/peppermint-oil/.

"Red Clover." n.d. Oregon Clover Commission. Accessed Sept. 28, 2022. https://www.oregonclover.org/pages/redclover.html.

"Sleep Basics." 2020. Cleveland Clinic, Dec. 7, 2020. https://my.clevelandclinic.org/health/articles/12148-sleep-basics.

"The Bioavailability of Different Forms of Vitamin C (Ascorbic Acid)". n.d. *Linus Pauling Institute*. Oregon State University. Accessed Dec. 5, 2021. http://lpi.oregonstate.edu/infocenter/vitamins/vitaminC/vitCform.html.

"The Truth About Glutathione". n.d. Accessed Oct. 27, 2021. https://edu.emersonecologics.com/2019/02/26/the-truth-about-glutathione-absorption/.

"Vis." n.d. Merriam Webster Dictionary, Accessed April 08, 2021. https://www.merriam-webster.com/dictionary/vis.

"What Happens to Your Body When You Quit Smoking?" n.d. *WebMD*. Accessed Sept. 2, 2021. https://www.webmd.com/smoking-cessation/what-happens-body-quit-smoking.

Image Attributions

2 Gas Exchange in the Lungs: bigstockphoto.com/image-367775671/

4 The Lymphatic: Systembigstockphoto.com/image-186011071

5 The Heart: bigstockphoto.com/image-397774385

6 The Circulatory System: bigstockphoto.com/image-412024246

8 Qigong: bigstockphoto.com/image-236148940

10 The Liver: freepik.com/free-vector/human-digestive-system_23816007.htm

11 The Kidneys: freepik.com/free-photo/woman-with-illuminated-kidneys_923797.htm

12 The Gastrointestinal System: freepik.com/free-vector/human-digestive-system_23816007.htm

13 The Skin: bigstockphoto.com/image-410453251

14 The Adrenals: bigstockphoto.com/image-222589453

15 The Thyroid: bigstockphoto.com/image-366447559

16 Nerve Cells: freepik.com/premium-photo/active-nerve-cells_6195725.htm

17 The Brain and Spine: bigstockphoto.com/image-430607117

18 Spinal Nerves: bigstockphoto.com/image-432374807

19 The Peripheral Nerves: bigstockphoto.com/image-451749909

20 The GI Tract: bigstockphoto.com/image-457956571

21 The Bones and Muscles: bigstockphoto.com/image-251380

22 Lymphatic Massage Chart: bigstockphoto.com/image-411814843

About the Author

Eli Camp, ND, DHANP, VNMI is a Naturopathic doctor who earned her medical degree from the Southwest College of Naturopathic Medicine in Tempe, AZ. She graduated in 2005 and established a private practice in New Hampshire. Her early years of practice were spent working with a large number of autistic children, many of whom were vaccine damaged. In addition to the autistic patient population, Dr. Camp has worked with hundreds of people to help them find a way to a better state of health. One of the early lessons she learned as a doctor was that each person has an individual capacity for making changes in their life, changes needed to establish the conditions of health. In her perspective, creating 100% optimal health is not only incredibly hard for most people it is not necessary to see great benefits. She uses the approach that it is far better and more successful to help people become healthy enough so that they watch symptoms disappear and feel better. She has worked with hundreds of people who smoke helping them to support their body, stimulate healing and enjoy a better quality of life.

Dr. Camp has written several books, including, *The Unvaccinated Child: A Treatment Guide for Parents and Caregivers* and *Homeopathy: A Foundational Approach*. She lectures across the country at numerous health conferences, public school districts and to the community in general regarding the topics of health and the practice of homeopathy. She serves as a preceptor for students from various fields of healthcare and as a mentor, consultant and coach to other Naturopathic Doctors to help them establish and become successful in private practice. Her memberships include the Oklahoma Association of Naturopathic Physicians (OKANP), the Homeopathic Academy of Naturopathic Physicians (HANP) and the Naturopathic Medicine Institute (NMI). In addition to membership, Dr. Camp currently serves on the Board of the NMI.

Several years ago, Dr. Camp and her family made a radical life change. They sold their home in Norman, OK, in a nice suburban neighborhood, and purchased land to become homesteaders. Her idea was to offer people an opportunity to join them as they created a new way of living life, one congruent with traditional Cherokee lifeways. Most days you can find her, her husband, Brian, and their adopted grandchildren, Brian and Sophia, and many volunteers digging in the garden, chasing ducks and chickens, chopping wood, canning and preserving food, foraging, tapping trees and so much more.

Dr. Camp believes we must be the change we wish to see in the world. So many of us did not learn these ways from our parents because they did not learn them from theirs. It is time to change this by relearning and passing on how to live with the land, produce food, and leave behind a better situation than the one we found.

Books by Vital Health Publishing

The Unvaccinated Child: A Treatment Guide for Parents and Caregivers

Guía para el cuidado natural de tus hijos

Homeopathy: A Foundational Approach

Smoke Rings: When everyone says not to but you want to anyway.

Fishkeeping For Kids by Brian Conway